The Portable Medical Mentor

.

Larry D. Florman, M.D.

The Portable Medical Mentor

Training Success

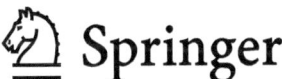 Springer

Larry D. Florman, M.D.
Division of Plastic Surgery
University of Louisville School of Medicine
Louisville, KY, USA

ISBN 978-3-319-09851-7   ISBN 978-3-319-09852-4 (eBook)
DOI 10.1007/978-3-319-09852-4
Springer Cham Heidelberg New York Dordrecht London

Library of Congress Control Number: 2014948340

Springer is part of Springer Science+Business Media (www.springer.com)

To Sadie, Nathan, Phyllis, Tammy, Jeffrey, and Sandy, my mentors for eternity.

Author's Note to Foreword

This forward written by Hiram C. Polk, M.D., and Kelly M. McMasters, M.D., Ph.D., is, with very minor changes, a reproduction of the foreword that Dr. Polk so graciously and expertly wrote in 2004 for the predecessor to this book entitled "*Portable Surgical Mentors: A Handbook of Protocol for Interns and Residents in Surgery*."

His words and thoughts 10 years ago are even more relevant today. Read their learned views very carefully. They will be just as salient 10, 20, 30 years from now.

Foreword

Precipitous and precarious change has become the norm in American medicine since this manual's first edition. Accomplishing the only stages of your education as a physician is occurring on a perpetually shifting stage. It is not just payment, access, quality, and mutual respect; patient expectations for uniformity of perfect care and services are greater than are applied to any other profession or industry.

This unprecedented change massively influences the domain of medical education. Whether one chooses to identify this with clinical training at the beginning of the third year of medical school or the completion of the seventh or eighth year of super-specialty training, many of the same issues and concerns apply. The transition from a scientifically oriented student to a real doctor is both fraught with hazard and consumes thousands of hours. Becoming a real doctor is fueled in many respects in the light of what most American patients expect their doctors to be. This marvelous, concise book is aimed precisely at helping you bridge that gap.

We have witnessed a decline in career choices, but now a reversal of that decline has occurred with a renewed growth of interest in careers in all of the specialties. Studies on workforce or old-fashioned manpower as it were continue to show that there is a growing demand for specialty services in America. Depending on where you live, it may be highly specialty oriented or nearer to "old-fashioned" general practice.

While the most dramatic of these issues are best understood in the traditional format of orderly training in a specialty in the USA, many of these concerns are international and apply irrespective of national boundaries or specialty. In fact, as an example, with a steadily important portion of the American medical trainee population being educated overseas, a book such as this has a very special and renewed value. The core competencies mandated for training in all specialties focus upon the following:

1. Patient care
2. Medical knowledge
3. Practice-based learning and improvement
4. Interpersonal and communication skills
5. Professionalism
6. Systems-based practice

These competencies reflect not only the old order of wisdom, skill, and knowledge in patient care, but also a new order related to communicating our understanding of the health system under which we attempt to work, especially the need for ongoing, and even increased professionalism. In earlier years, professionalism was taught in a simple apprentice matter by observing other physicians who had learned from their mentors, across generations, about the ethical, the courteous, the considerate, and the humane practice of medicine. This book admirably helps inculcate the above qualities in the student of medicine.

Because of many issues impacting training, particularly the shortened duty hours, opportunities for this type of observed interaction are now significantly less frequent; the nature of the American health system and its scheme for reimbursement have compacted the formerly leisurely, warm, and personal opportunity that should mark each patient contact. It is ironic and also appropriate that professionalism to some degree is now going to be taught in a classroom and or read in a book. One could find few better aids to crossing such an important chasm than this particular manual. Indeed, there is not a single anecdote or truism noted in this treatise that I have not observed, for better or worse, and would have wished to teach so clearly.

It is no accident that this is the product of a lifetime of experiences from an ethical practice within a specialty located in a hospital and associated with a major, old, but characteristically mid-American School of Medicine. There is no need to comment on such an overtly practical content, but communication involves direct personal interface with patients and all other healthcare professionals. This is a reminder that "thank you" can always close any kind of contact with any of your professional and personal colleagues to your advantage.

The life of a physician does involve communication throughout an evermore modern healthcare system which on occasion does become disruptive in and of itself. The physician's conduct in the hospital and in his office is special points of worthy attention, since they set the ambience for the conduct of the team that surrounds him. There are now dramatic reports of the soothing role of teamwork in the medical profession and those in which the stage is set for the highest quality care with a minimum opportunity for adverse events for the patient's safety and well-being.

The doctor's office is another case in point, and the new physician should especially be reminded that timeliness is especially appreciated. If one is running late for very legitimate reasons, apologizing for your tardiness, and even offering to discount or eliminate the bill in the office always puts that kind of unpleasant interaction in a more positive and generous light.

Again, one needs to be reminded that patients do not always hear and/or remember what you have said, and it may be helpful to clarify and expand some of these discussions, especially when concerning prognosis or directions taking medications. We should do this with another family member present and be certain to briefly describe the nature of that discussion in the patient's chart.

"Compliance" has become a dirty word within medicine, but it simply means what most of us for multiple generations have known and accepted: Write in the chart in a legible, accurate, and timely way exactly what you have done, what you have said, and what you expect as a result of that interaction. As a matter of fact, it may also be helpful to indicate what progress you expect in the period before your next set of rounds, or before the next office visit.

It has long been my thought that physicians who speak well, often think well, and being called upon to speak clearly and with a minimum of medical jargon reflect favorably on the doctor and all of his or her contacts. This especially includes presentations at rounds and in quality improvement conferences, which now certainly characterize the teamwork as a mark of contemporary medicine. Indeed, there was an era in which the solo practitioner was the prototype American physician. Now you are part of a team from the moment you begin your internship, often until you conclude your practice 35 years later, with the legitimate and ethical lifestyle of a hopefully closely knit group practice, defining exactly what one can do. The availability of a physician is essential, and one must never be less than vigilant in ensuring that your patients who are ill have the opportunity to reach you or a qualified and informed individual legally and ethically associated with you. The most difficult part of the 80-h duty week has not been contriving schedules, identifying nurse practitioners, and/or creating night floats, but in the actual "hand-off" to doctor A to doctor B to doctor C. Everyone is alert to these issues that have posed unanticipated and unforeseen consequences, and we are all working towards methods to make those evermore safe and evermore efficient.

The balance within one's life is an important undertaking, and this means refreshing your professionally fatigued mind and body with relationships with family and friends that are healthy and, indeed, renew you to resume your active medical practice.

Any foreword is intended to be a cameo of what the content of a handbook may be and should be. The fact that this book has been developed by a person with a lifetime success in practice who has now moved towards a full-time teaching role for new generations, not just for surgical specialists such as himself, but for the newest and most naïve third-year medical student, adds a substance of freshness, vitality, and interest. It clearly can be useful and will be the sort of thing that stays close in your hand and at your side across your early years in training and in practice.

Hiram C. Polk
Department of Surgery
School of Medicine
University of Louisville
Louisville, KY, USA
June, 2014

Kelly M. Mcmasters, M.D., PhD.
Chairman, Department of Surgery
School of Medicine
University of Louisville
Louisville, KY, USA
June, 2014

Preface

"What lies behind us and what lies before us are small matters compared to what lies within us."

— Ralph Waldo Emerson

This book has been lovingly written to aid our young colleagues, who by their choice of pursuing an education in medicine have, in fact, dedicated the rest of their lives to compassion, to study, to knowledge, and to humanity. The purpose of this book is to inculcate the discipline necessary for them to successfully care for the patient and to teach this discipline to others. This is not a medical book per se. The subject may at first elude the young student, intern, resident, or fellow. The principles will ultimately intertwine with their lives so tightly that they will rapidly and joyfully witness in themselves the metamorphosis of the classroom student into the polished physician.

A prevailing theme throughout this book, regardless of the stage of training, is that being the best physician that one can be will most certainly lead to career success.

My best regards and hopes for an exciting and rewarding journey.

Louisville, KY, USA   Larry D. Florman, M.D.

Acknowledgements

To acknowledge but a few would be a disservice to everyone who gave of themselves so willingly and enthusiastically towards the completion of this book. But, disservice I must do to a few in order to emphasize the wonderful contributions of the following people:

Hiram C. Polk, Jr., M.D., and Kelly M. McMasters, M.D., Ph.D., for their constant concern, encouragement, and flawless expertise.

Jason Smith, M.D., Ph.D., for conceiving and playing a most important role in developing the chapter on "Going in to Practice."

Russell W. Farmer, M.D., who succinctly aided in writing the chapters on Insurance, Managed Care, Electronic Medical Record, and Social Media.

Erica R. Sutton, M.D., who masterfully aided in writing the chapter on Teaching and Learning. And, who was a constant source of advice and encouragement to the author.

Ms. Carlene L. Petty, a wonderful artist, for her superb caricatures.

Ms. Margaret A. Abby, for her encouragement and masterful editorial skills.

Contents

The Author

Larry D. Florman M.D. was born and raised in Pittsburgh, Pennsylvania. He attended undergraduate school at the Youngstown University in Ohio and medical school at the University of Louvain in Belgium. He completed a rotating internship at the Queen Elizabeth Hospital in Montreal; general surgery residency at the Beth Israel Medical Center in New York City; and a residency in otolaryngology at the Manhattan Eye, Ear, and Throat Hospital in New York City. This was followed by a residency in plastic and reconstructive surgery at the University of Louisville in Kentucky. He is board certified in Plastic and Reconstructive Surgery as well as Otolaryngology-Head and Neck Surgery.

Following 28 years of private practice and teaching as a clinical instructor, in 2002, Dr. Florman ended his private practice in the traditional sense and assumed the title of Assistant Professor of Surgery at the University of Louisville School of Medicine, where he has been training young surgeons to be plastic surgeons and otolaryngologists. He now limits his private practice to aesthetic and reconstructive surgery of the nose.

Dr. Florman's wife Phyllis is an attorney, arbitrator, and mediator. They have three children: a daughter who is the director of marketing at a large Chicago firm, a son who is a neurosurgeon, and another son who is a transplant surgeon. When not busy teaching, he builds and flies experimental airplanes, restores automobiles, tinkers in electronics, is an amateur radio operator, gardens, and worries about his eight grandchildren.

Chapter 1
Introduction

*"By three methods we may learn wisdom. First,
by reflection, which is noblest, second, by imitation,
which is easiest? and third by experience, which is
the bitterest?"*

— Confucius

Training in medicine is a lifelong process or should we refer to it as a "journey." The journey does not begin with medical school and end at retirement, but commences at some point in one's life when that individual realizes that he has the ability, the drive, and the self-assurance to actually make a difference in caring for the health and welfare of fellow human beings.

It is the intent of this "handbook" to encourage and demonstrate to physicians-to-be and to newly ordained physicians that they can and must be the very best that they can be. Nobody believes that there are "born doctors." In fact, the process of becoming a physician not only involves a formal education, but a veritable lifelong personality change. One must begin to think and behave as a medical professional, all the while learning the principles and techniques of their chosen specialty. Some will not find it easy to achieve this balance, as there are many ingrained habits and external influences that may lead to resistance of the change that must take place. In medical school one attains all of the essential

L.D. Florman, *The Portable Medical Mentor:
Training Success*, DOI 10.1007/978-3-319-09852-4_1,
© Springer International Publishing Switzerland 2015

book knowledge but only a smattering of the behavioral changes that are necessary to fulfill their obligations. In the past, these rules of conduct have been forced upon the fledgling physician by those directly superior to him. Sometimes this system would work, and often it would not, leaving the apprentice physician to move up in the ladder of the educational process alone, instilling in himself concepts in behavior that could sometimes be erroneous, unhealthy, detrimental to patients, detrimental to other house staffs, and not least, damaging to his remaining years in the practice of medicine.

When compared with other countries, the American method of training young physicians is very "generous," not as demanding, and yet more thorough. "Generous" means the house staffer in the USA is given an ever-increasing role and authority in the care of patients in his charge. This graduated responsibility not only shifts some of the burden of patient care from the attending physician, but also offers the young physician increasing responsibilities that are necessary to pursue and to teach our profession correctly.

The demands made of the contemporary house staffer are truly not as enormous as in the past. The 80-h workweek rule can be strongly debated either way. However, in the end, it guarantees that the physician-in-training will work fewer hours than his predecessors, have less time with direct patient contact, less time under the direct tutelage of his experienced elders, and less time developing relationships with other professionals. Today, residents will work until the 80 h is reached. Students will work even less. Then, the remainder of the process will consist of self-help. The author has attempted, with the help of his mentors, to record the experiences of students, interns, residents, fellows, physicians, teachers, professors, sons, daughters, husbands, wives, parents, friends, and fellow travelers. The sacred adage that "experience is the best teacher" is as true as ever when applied to the learning and the practice of medicine in general, and the specialties in particular. We have learned what works and what does not.

If one were to distill in the reader the essentials derived from the "portable mentor," or any mentor, the most important would be:

Be **honest** (with yourself and others).
Be **kind** (with yourself and others) (it costs you nothing)
Be **humble**.

In choosing medicine, you have agreed to dedicate yourself to these principles. Hopefully by reading this book, you will ease your journey into being the very best that you can be. The goal of this book is to offer you a "leg up" on the art of becoming the best student that you can be, and by creating in you the best student as is possible. There will be no attempt to teach you medicine, per se. Perhaps many of the items that are discussed in this book may seem trivial and superfluous. They are not! Some of the qualities that you will read about may not occur with the house staff at your institution, but it would be very difficult for anyone to disagree with the principles that you are about to read. Even if you do not immediately agree with the need for them, try them! Force yourself to weave some of these concepts into your every waking moment.

Several cleanup items to consider:

1. Quite arbitrarily, the author has elected to make this text unisex. All references of gender should be viewed as interchangeable.
2. The author has strategically placed *in italics* some anecdotal tales, sometimes to make a point, sometimes just because it is a good story. All of the stories are true. Of course, the names have been changed to protect the guilty.
3. Each institution has its own rules and its own ways of doing things. We would not be pretentious enough to suggest that you follow our way to the exclusion of your medical school or training institution.
4. The contents of this book are meant for the young medical student, resident, intern, and fellow, regardless of his/her future goals in medicine.

5. You might suggest to your spouse, your significant other, or your mother to read this book. It will demonstrate to each of them what is expected of you, what you are going through, and the amazing commitment that you have made.
6. Throughout this book the author has endeavored to use "we" instead of "I" (when referring to the author). In fact, the writing of this book has been made possible by the collaborative effort of every individual and event that the author has experienced in his medical career. In your efforts and successes in training and in the practice of medicine try the "we" thing. After all, the successes are always a collaborative effort. For the failures, take the hit and use "I."

Chapter 2
Mentors/Advisors

> *"My chief want in life is someone who shall make me do what I can."*
>
> — Ralph Waldo Emerson

This could very well be for you the most important chapter of this book.

Webster's Dictionary defines "mentor" as "*A wise and faithful counselor or monitor*." It defines "adviser" as "one who gives advice." Many medical students, interns, residents, and fellows have an advisor, somebody to make suggestions to them based on that person's knowledge of the trainee, and knowledge of the field for which they are giving advice. Advice is very often handed out as the result of a request, or sometimes voluntarily with the idea of making a useful suggestion. Everybody has at least one adviser. Perhaps an advisor for "how should I study for anatomy" is not the same as the one for "what elective rotation should I take." It is not unusual to have several advisers. In medical school an adviser is often appointed to you. Sometimes you will seek his/her advice, and sometimes you will not. Sometimes the advice will be the result of an extensive experience and sometimes it will be the result of no experience with the question at all. There are so many quotes and sayings about advice and advisers, and most of them are not complimentary. That is not to say that there are not some very good advisers with some

L.D. Florman, *The Portable Medical Mentor: Training Success*, DOI 10.1007/978-3-319-09852-4_2,
© Springer International Publishing Switzerland 2015

very good advice. Ask your friends and older colleagues who you should go to for good, reliable, educated, advice on a particular subject.

Mentor 3 was the son of Heracles and Asopis. In his old age Mentor 3 was the wise and trusted adviser to Odysseus who placed Mentor and Odysseus' foster-brother Eumaeus in charge of his son Telemachus, and also of Odysseus' palace, when Odysseus left to lead the Trojan War.

When Athena visited Telemachus she took the disguise of Mentor 3 to hide herself from the suitors of Telemachus's mother Penelope. As Mentor 3, the goddess encouraged Telemachus to stand up against the suitors and go abroad to find out what happened to his father. Mentor 3 was indeed a wonderful adviser to the young man. There is a thought that he also was quite close to Penelope.

Because of Mentor 3's relationship with Telemachus, and the disguised Athena's encouragement and practical plans for dealing with personal dilemmas, the personal name *Mentor* has been adopted in English as a term meaning someone who imparts wisdom to, and shares knowledge with, a less experienced colleague.

The old system of medical education in Europe was for a physician to personally teach a young student everything from the basic sciences to the details of his specialty. Usually the student lived in his mentor's home. Not infrequently he ended up marrying the mentor's daughter. This was true mentorship. Today, mentoring takes on many forms. But, the common element is an unwritten dedication on the part of the mentor to see that his mentored not only succeeds, but also thrives.

The mentor/mentored relationship is one of thoughtful, caring, compassionate attention. One can have more than one mentor, or different ones for different levels of training. A mentor can have more than one mentored. For the student at any level, the mentor connection just happens. It cannot be pre-programmed. The student becomes so enamored of a prospective mentor that the relationship just seems to grow and flourish. The mentor sees in a student the opportunity for that student to achieve greatness with the proper direction. The mentor/mentored relationship seems almost chemical.

So, how do you get an advisor? If an advisor is not appointed to you, or you don't care for your present or assigned advisor, or if you want a different advisor, or if you need an additional advisor, just ask. If you have no idea who should be giving you advice, ask your friends, your seniors, your professors, and your chiefs. Then, do it face to face, not by e-mail or telephone. Be specific in your request. With the proper chemistry, this could end up as a mentor relationship.

So, how do you get a mentor? This is no easy task. In fact, this is not at all a task. It is not a formal liaison. The word "mentor" may not ever be said. It is just a feeling on your part, and on the part of the mentor. You may have a mentor and not know it. Someone who is quietly watching over you, delicately steering you in the right direction, and ready to take on a very active role in your career if you wave a flag. A long time after, perhaps years, you may suddenly realize that at some distinct time you had a mentor, and you will drop him/her a note of recognition and appreciation, or just a Christmas card.

Chapter 3
The Transition: Part 1

"My grandfather once told me that there were two kinds of people: those who do the work and those who take the credit. He told me to try to be in the first group; there was much less competition."

— Indira Gandhi

During the clinical years in medical school, you are gradually becoming a physician. Then you are an intern, resident, and fellow. Veritably overnight, you must now devote your entire being to the profession that you have chosen. This part of your education can be very daunting, and, if not taken seriously, can affect the rest of your career or even put a sudden stop to it. Whether you like it or not, once you receive, or have received that diploma, and your family and friends address you as "doctor," your life changes forever. If it does not change, then you are doing something wrong. Remember, this change must start to occur the very first time you are exposed to a patient, or better yet, before.

There are certain conventions by which you must now abide. You must permit your education, your experiences, graduation day, and the rest of your career to blend in seamlessly with this new life. You are now a physician with all of the powerful properties, attributes, and responsibilities that accompany the title. Do not resist your new level. Do not rebel against it. Do not believe for one moment that things

L.D. Florman, *The Portable Medical Mentor:*
Training Success, DOI 10.1007/978-3-319-09852-4_3,
© Springer International Publishing Switzerland 2015

will be the same in your life. Rise to the occasion. Here are several guidelines to live by, and live by them you must:

1. ***You now LIVE IN A GLASS HOUSE***. Get used to it quickly. Your every action will be noted and scrutinized by family, friends, and the public. Curtains on the windows will not shield you from the prying eye. The person who sees you do something foolish (or courageous) today may be your patient, car mechanic, or banker tomorrow.

   If you have had one too many margaritas at a party last night, might not someone believe that you will be a menace in the operating room tomorrow? If you drive home after those three beers, might not one believe that you lack good judgment? If you smoked something mood elevating or ingested something mind altering, might not a close friend, 5 years later, who, in need of you in the emergency room, question whether you had a little puff before coming to sew up his child or take care of his mother's diabetic shock?

   How about the waiter to whom you acted like a positive jerk, and whose sister works in housekeeping at the hospital, and also whose brother cuts the grass for your chairman? People talk.

   Your entire life is an open book, whether or not you like it. News of misguided behavior travels fast and is often quickly exaggerated. It is just about impossible to extract yourself from it. Make your behavior as exemplary as you would wish upon your children.

   The medical community all around the country is quite small. Everybody talks. Your ability to acquire a great or any residency position will be dependent on many factors, notably, grades, scores, clinical evaluations, letter of recommendation, and the infamous interview. A good performance in all of the above is important. However, one negative parameter of your education or personal life could very well undo all of your hard work. So, why have a negative in an item or items that you have complete control over, and that are so easy to avoid?

2. ***BE HUMBLE***. You have earned the privilege of being a physician. You now have achieved an expertise that very

few enjoy. Being a physician does not necessarily mean that you are a better person than others, or that you deserve special consideration, or that you are higher on the evolutionary scale.

Each of us is a traveler on the same road of life. If you are a better physician, then there is a better nurse, trash collector, or stock broker. Only allow your pride to guide you to be the best that you can be, not to be better than anyone else. Consider the following true story:

I like to consider myself a humble person. I recently attended a high school reunion. I joined a small crowd having drinks. Many recognized me, and I recognized very few of them. As everybody was taking turns telling of their achievements in life, it came around to me.
"So, what do you do?"
I gave my usual retort, "I work in a hospital."
"Well, what do you do in the hospital?"
"I work in surgery."
"Well, exactly what do you do in surgery?" asked another of my old classmates, expecting me to say that I cleaned the floors or changed the light bulbs. After hearing of the multitude of successes of this small group, lawyers, businessmen, psychologists, and internists, I said with a wry smirk,
"I am a plastic surgeon."
One said, "Yeah, sure!" The others bowed their heads, and the group immediately broke up and reassembled on the other side of the room.

Humility is a characteristic that you can learn. Closely observe people who you really like, regardless of profession. If you like them, then most likely one of their leading characteristics is humility.

3. ***BE RESPECTFUL* and courteous to everyone that you encounter**, regardless of profession or station in life. It is better and easier to be respectful than to treat someone as though they were not there, or didn't count, or are beneath you. Why not? What does it cost you? How can it be wrong

to be just plain "nice"? People surrounding you will note your behavior, and might even call you "nice" by the way you treat others.

4. **Be aware that *MORALITY and ETHICS* have a strong interplay when it comes to the practice of medicine**. A lack of either may get you into the kind of trouble that could follow you for the rest of your life. Certain actions you take will change your life in a major, detrimental fashion:

   • A felony conviction of any kind will most likely result in your dismissal from medical school or residency, the permanent revocation of your license to practice medicine in every state, or, at the very least, rejection by credentialing committees of hospitals and malpractice insurance companies. There is a national data bank which these organizations are privy to, and they do check them frequently.

   • Any conviction or revelation of drug or alcohol abuse could relieve you of your training position, or at the least necessitates your attending remediation in the form of governmental programs. This will have to be reported for the rest of your career.

   • Any conviction for illicit prescribing of medication will prevent you from completing medical school, or will certainly get you fired from your residency position. These will virtually be impossible to reclaim where you are training or anywhere in the USA.

   • Any lies, mistruths, or partial truths of any kind on your medical applications (training programs, hospitals, state licensing boards, insurance applications, etc.) will eventually surface and cause you grief for the rest of your career.

   It goes without saying that your moral values must be beyond reproach.

5. ***COMPASSION* is a concept that is impossible to teach, but quite easy to teach oneself**. If anybody is asked if they are compassionate, they will answer in the affirmative. Everybody will have a slightly different definition of the

word. If asked to identify the last time you demonstrated an act of compassion, you will have a difficult time pinning it down, or verbalizing it.

Compassion is easy to learn. You teach yourself. Consciously show an act of compassion at least once a day. Force yourself. It might feel strange to you. Hold a patient's hand. Physically touch them. Ask them if they want another blanket, a drink of water, the door closed. Sit on the bed when you talk to them. Hold the door open for the cleaning lady. Ask the nurse how her baby is doing. Compassion comes in an infinite number of forms. It can be as minimal as a pat on the back, a certain tilt of the head, or an "ah" at the right time. It can also take the form of driving a patient home from the clinic, buying a candy bar for a homeless man, or shedding a tear at a dying patient's bedside.

An interviewer gave the following scenario to a medical student applying for a residency in neurosurgery. Your trauma team is called to the emergency room at 3:00 AM to see a 21-year-old lady in an MVA. As the team enters the room, the neurosurgeons are leaving. The chief neurosurgery resident tells your chief residency to "forget it," she is a goner. The right side of her head is crushed. She is not a candidate for surgery and she is essentially dead but her heart is beating. She is intubated but not on a respirator. The chief trauma surgery resident points to you the medical student, and says "stay in the room. We are going to see another patient. When her heart stops beating, call me so that I can call my attending and tell him there has been a death on the service." No, there is no family available. Everybody leaves the room and you are alone with the patient. What are you going to do?

The interviewer has been given several different responses. Examine the patient and make sure that she is going to die? When nobody is looking go to the medicine cabinet and get some blood pressure drugs? Call the attending and tell him you don't like this job? Refuse? If you know what to do in this instance, would you have done it? Now you know what COMPASSION is.

Or, compassion can be crying with a patient or family member, taking your Saturday off to attend a free clinic, or … hold the hand and talk to an unconscious 21-year-old lady whose head is crushed and has only moments to live.

Give it a try. Do one act of compassion at least once a day. You will rapidly determine that it is very easy. Yes, it might take a few extra seconds out of your busy schedule, or it could take several minutes or hours. It might even cost you a couple of dollars. You will rapidly determine that it feels good to you, and that you will bask in the afterglow.

Be assured that true acts of compassion do not go unnoticed. Patients, family, friends, nurses, students, residents, attendings, chiefs, and many others will not forget you.

Chapter 4
Attire

"I'm tired of all this nonsense about beauty being only skin deep. That's deep enough. What do you want, an adorable pancreas?"

—Jean Kerr

Dress codes are institution specific, which means that most institutions have a dress code, but it is usually nonspecific. For students in the preclinical years an upgrade in clothes from college is in order, but not mandatory. However, you will make a better impression on your professors and colleagues. Dress nicely. Dress appropriately.

During the clinical years when you will be seeing patients if only as an observer, you must start looking like a doctor. Dress as well as the most senior resident, that is, if he is dressed well. Remember, you will impress your attendings and residents alike.

During these years you are on a mission. You are on a mission to impress. Residents and attendings are easily impressed, and more easily unimpressed. Regardless of your future goals, you will need these people to speak well of you when it comes time to evaluate you and write letters for your residency applications. Remember, you live in a very small community. Reports of shabbiness travel.

L.D. Florman, *The Portable Medical Mentor:*
Training Success, DOI 10.1007/978-3-319-09852-4_4,
© Springer International Publishing Switzerland 2015

In residency, dress professionally. Most likely you will begin your career by dressing quite well, and you will certainly impress everyone, even your fellow, slovenly dressed interns and residents (and some attendings). After a short period of time, you will see exactly what you can get away with, and in an effort to make your life easier, you will "sink" to the unwritten, house-staff invented, less than crisp, form of attire. Gentlemen, keep your necktie cinched up. Check it frequently. A chief, attending, or hospital administrator would prefer nothing more than to see their house staff appearing very professional. This simply means a clean shirt, perhaps a nice tie, clean white lab coat, shined shoes (never clogs or sandals and never flip-flops), and socks. Regardless of how your attendings and the chief are dressed, this is the way you should dress.

Your professors and attendings will remember you if you are dressed well, or poorly. They will think better of you if you are well dressed. They might even write you a better letter of recommendation when the time comes. They will certainly feel better about you when it comes time to evaluate your performance. Think, who would you want coming in to your mother's hospital room (Fig. 4.1)?

Dressing for your new station in life can often divert unwanted attention away from other inadequacies. Why not take every opportunity to impress your superiors and your patients? For your patients it is sort of a form of reassurance that you are the professional that you portend to be. For your superiors it is sort of a form of reassurance that you are the professional that you portend to be. It does not take much effort, and it will reassure everybody that surrounds you of your professional competence, even if that assurance is not really merited. You may even impress yourself with how well you clean up, and it could very well even start a positive trend among your fellow workers.

The stethoscope is not an article of clothing. Students, interns, residents, fellows, and attendings wear their stethoscope in and on different parts of their body for varying reasons. The most usual reason is to impress. It impresses

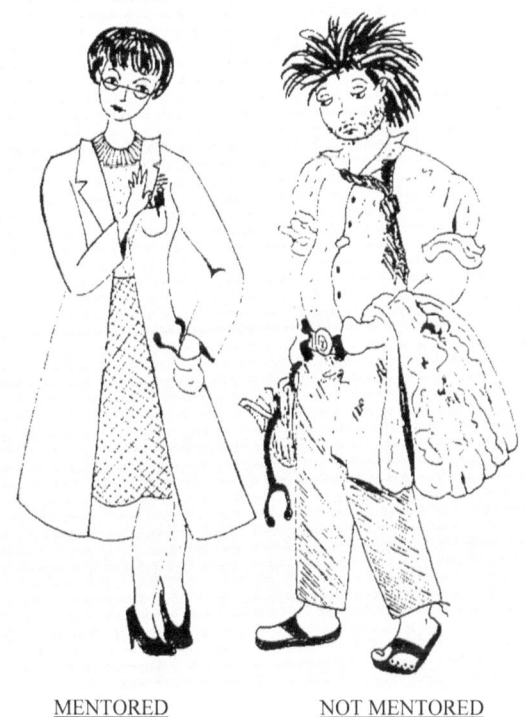

MENTORED   NOT MENTORED

FIG. 4.1.   Proper and improper attire

nobody. The author has seen young doctors and students with their stethoscope around their necks in supermarkets, gas stations, and sitting at tables in restaurants. When not in use keep your stethoscope in your pocket (Fig. 4.2).

A word about grooming should not have to be said at this point, but we have seen too many ungroomed or poorly groomed house staffs walking the hospital wards. This seems to be a holdover from medical school days. It is very noticeable and does not impress anyone. Comb your hair. Have your hair groomed regularly. If you wear other facial hair (beard, goatee, etc.), then it should appear neat. Better yet, do not wear it. Keep your face shaved. If you were on call the

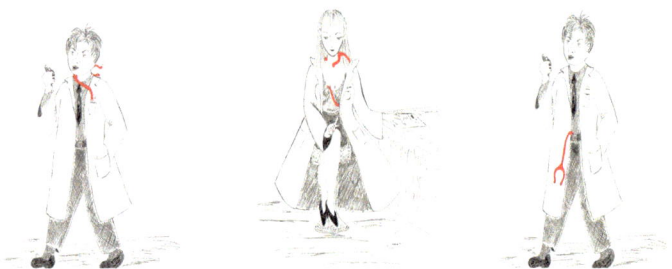

Fɪɢ. 4.2. Wear your badge of honor in your heart, not wrapped around your neck

night before and must visit patients in the morning, then wake up 3 min earlier and shave. Get your teeth cleaned regularly; nobody likes to see your winning smile with a mouth full of tarter. Keep your fingernails trimmed and clean at all times. Patients and patient's families often pay attention to the fingernails of physicians.

Scrubs should not be worn in the street. Some institutions turn a blind eye to this practice, and some absolutely forbid it. Not only does it raise the question of the cleanliness of the operating room environment, but also you will actually start to walk into the operating room with those same street scrubs. Conversely, you could be accused of spreading hospital germs to the public on the street. It only takes 1 min to change your clothes. For obvious reasons, do not wear scrubs home. If you must walk out of the operating suite with scrubs on, you must wear a white lab coat. Never walk out of the operating room with a mask, cap, or booties. It does not impress anyone.

In the hospital, wear clean pants, a clean shirt of any color, and a necktie. A white lab coat is preferred; however, it must always be clean. Always wear socks. Absolutely no sandals are allowed.

If you have been called to the chief's office, wear a blue or black blazer.

The same scrub rules apply to women in every instance. The same white lab coat rules apply. A skirt or a long dress is definitely acceptable in place of pants. A pants suit can take the place of a white lab coat. No visible body piercing, except for one (preferable) or two ear piercings, and of course, only those body piercings as mandated by religious customs. It gives no reassurance to a patient or their family to have a doctor come in to the hospital room with a diamond-studded post in their eyebrow, lip, or nose. If at all possible cover up your tattoos when seeing patients.

You dressed well for your interview for this position. Consider every day of your life as an interview. You will be graded or scored for the rest of your career.

Chapter 5
The Little Black Book

Order marches with weighty and measured strides.
Disorder is always in a hurry.

—Napoleon Bonaparte

How often have you observed a more senior resident in his clean, pressed, white lab coat, with his pens and little flashlights arranged neatly in the lapel pocket, his tie precisely placed, his hospital badge appropriately and very visibly showing, his stethoscope just peeking out of his pocket so that everybody knows he is a doctor, searching among many different pieces of crumbled paper in his pockets? Medicine is a rather orderly avocation, and any hint of disorganization gives the overall impression of confusion and sloppiness, and can be dangerous. A device that helps you to organize your life and your job must be at your fingertips at all times.

In the past this consisted of a little 6- or 8-ring "black book" that would easily fit into your white jacket pocket. In the present, it is still the little 6- or 8-ring black book, but the electronic substitute is rapidly taking over. Historically, and currently, the drug companies and other purveyors of medical items and services have made the black books available at no cost to the house staff. They usually do not fulfill the need.

This little black book, whether electronic or traditional, should be used to store the information about your life and your job in an orderly fashion, and, at the same time, be easily

L.D. Florman, *The Portable Medical Mentor:*
Training Success, DOI 10.1007/978-3-319-09852-4_5,
© Springer International Publishing Switzerland 2015

accessible. Here are a few of the items that this portable medium must include:

- Calendar with as much detail as possible (meetings, schedules, rounds, holidays, vacations, birthdays, time off, deadlines, etc.).
- Names, addresses, phone numbers, cellular numbers, pager numbers, fax numbers, e-mail addresses of everyone you may possibly need to contact. Phone numbers of various hospitals, with extension numbers of frequently used departments (operating room, scheduling, nursing units, medical records, medical staff office, emergency department, pathology, X-ray, lab, etc.).
- Patient lists (annotated).
- A section for frequently used drugs, their doses, and special indications. Assuming that you will have a smartphone or electronic tablet, you should install the PDR (Physician's Desk Reference) app.
- A section dedicated to the idiosyncrasies of your attending staff.
- An appendix with conversion charts (metric/British), formulas, etc.
- There are great apps for medical drawing which could come in useful to better demonstrate areas of anatomy to patients and families.

It is essential to obtain a method for storing your affairs in some sort of orderly fashion. What will not work is crumbled pieces of paper or your brain.

You have at least three choices ... a PDA (personal digital assistant), a little ringed book (3, 4, or 8 ring), and a cell phone with areas for calendar and notes. There are pros and cons for each:

5.1   PDA

Pro

(a) Compact
(b) No pages to shuffle through or fall out

(c) Easily readable
(d) Calendar is very detailed (i.e., month, date, year, weekly, monthly, yearly)
(e) Can easily be downloaded to your PC
(f) Bulk information can be placed in PC and then down-loaded to PDA
(g) Alarms
(h) Never becomes bulky
(i) Could include a cellular phone all in one
(j) Ability to transfer information from one PDA to another PDA (patient lists, schedules, etc.)
(k) Possibility of downloading ACLS/CPR references, case tracking software, PDR, and digitized texts. Some hospitals are equipped to download patient lists, lab reports, etc., through their Wi-Fi network

Con

(a) Cost
(b) Important to back up information to PC on a regular basis
(c) Learning curve
(d) Graffiti not always accurate
(e) Some actions may take longer to get to
(f) Need to change batteries or charge
(g) HIPPA violations possible if lost or stolen.

5.2 Little Black Book

Pro

(a) Inexpensive
(b) Easier and quicker to access and view different sections
(c) Place to put extraneous papers
(d) Blank pages can be torn out and given to others
(e) No batteries needed, no downloads, no backup
(f) No limit on memory
(g) Easier to keep patient lists

Con

(a) Need something to write with
(b) Can get bulky
(c) Need to carry blank pages
(d) Pages can tear out
(e) No backup possible
(f) Not as "cool-looking" as PDA

Whatever you decide, you should make optimal use of your method. Do not be without it. Keep it up to date, rely on it, and use it. It will facilitate your life and make you appear more put together.

Chapter 6
Communications

> *"What we have here is a failure to communicate."*
>
> —From the film "Cool Hand Luke"

Speaking in the medical vernacular is important to effectively, succinctly, and accurately communicate with your colleagues. This subject will be discussed in subsequent chapters. In this chapter, the focus is on the methods for others to contact or communicate with you via overhead pages, pagers, cell phones, two-way radios, home telephones, text messages, and e-mails, and for you to communicate with them.

The availability of clear and immediate communications is very important for quality patient care, from the way that you appear to others to the smooth operation of the institution. Answer all overhead pages immediately. Never be complacent when screening numbers on cell phones or pagers in order to determine the importance of the messages before answering them. The usual, frequent, benign call may be the one instance when it is a very urgent message. Frequently check the condition of your electronic device. Make sure that the batteries are new or fully charged. Know where spare batteries are located for immediate replacement. Charge your device every day, even if it has a 36-h standby time. Frequently check that the ringer is turned on and is loud enough. If possible, have it ring and vibrate at the same time.

L.D. Florman, *The Portable Medical Mentor:*   25
Training Success, DOI 10.1007/978-3-319-09852-4_6,
© Springer International Publishing Switzerland 2015

What follows is a review of the modern means of communications:

6.1   Overhead Page

Very unreliable.

Every hospital has an overhead paging system, but this form of communication is unreliable, as it does not reach certain areas of the hospital, and it is not always clearly audible. It usually does not work in the operating rooms, the restrooms, the on-call rooms, or patient's rooms. Therefore, do not count on it. Never ask anyone to page you overhead. If you should receive an overhead page, you should check your pager or cell phone to ensure that the switch is turned on and the ringer is loud enough. Of course, respond immediately.

Most hospitals use the overhead page for emergency or urgent situations. There is often a coding system to these pages—such as "Code Blue 3rd floor toilets." When you are able you should take these seriously and aid the situation.

6.2   Digital or Numeric Pager

Very reliable.

Your institution will usually provide a pager for you at no cost. It will be the "monkey on your back" for at least the rest of your training. It is your duty and obligation to carry it with you, even when not on call. There is no telling when and where the boss (your chief, your mother, your wife) may be looking for you.

In the operating room, you should place the device on a table and alert the circulating nurse where it is located and what to do with it. There are usually several pagers on the table, so put a label on your pager so that the nurse knows to whom it belongs.

These are generally not rechargeable, so have a place to go for a battery change when indicated.

6.3   Cell Phone

Very reliable.

This is, of course, the gold standard of communications. But, only as good as the owner who pays attention to it. Some institutions provide cell phones to their house staff at no cost. Others demand them of the house staff and make you assume the cost. When not required, many house staffers will purchase one at their own expense, because it will make their lives easier. Regardless of who purchases one, make sure that you make good use of the special features such as the built-in phone book, speed dialing, calendar, and notes. There are some wonderful apps for the medical profession (Appendix A).

It may be considered impolite to talk on your cell phone while with groups of people, in restaurants, theaters, elevators, and in patient's rooms. It is against the law (HIPAA) to speak of patients by name or in any identifiable form within audible reach of the lay public. Password your cell phone. Check frequently that you have not missed a call or text message. Ideally, don't permit any call to go into voicemail, and if it does, respond as soon as practical. At home don't let the kids play with it, or the wife answer it.

6.4   Two-Way Radio

Some institutions provide this means of communications for certain physicians in strategic positions, such as for trauma surgeons, who must provide a quick response. Beware that the usable distance is short, and these instruments should not leave the hospital.

6.5   Home Telephone

Your home phone is not off limits to hospital business. Never put your home phone on "do not disturb." Never neglect answering the phone at any time or in any circumstance.

Do not screen your calls. Have a phone extension at your bedside. List your home phone number at the hospital switchboard. Make sure that all of your colleagues have your telephone number, pager number, and cell phone number in their little black book (Chap. 5.2). Remember that cell phone systems and pager systems do fail from time to time. You are obligated to always have a line of communications open to your colleagues and to the hospital. In certain medical situations and with certain patients there is nothing wrong with giving them your cell phone number.

This chapter would not be complete without a word about vacations, time away from home, and time off. It is essential that your senior resident knows how to reach you during your entire time in training. Leaving your phone number with the department secretary is necessary, but not good enough. A secretary does not work on the weekends or at night. If you will be away overnight or out of pager and cell phone range, an on-call house staff person must be able to reach you. Often you will know the patient best, which is why you can positively impact their care with your unique knowledge of their history. Residency is a 100 % of the time job/occupation.

6.6   E-Mail

E-mail is a wonderful means by which you can communicate with your colleagues in either a casual or formal setting. It must be kept in mind that the internet is not at all secure. Patient information or identifying characteristics should not be transmitted by means of an unsecured e-mail message. This could be a violation of HIPAA laws. Never communicate medical information or instructions to a patient by unsecured e-mail, notably because you will not know if they received the e-mail and/or who received the e-mail. Keep in mind that e-mails are discoverable by courts of law.

Regardless of the means, answer all of your calls immediately. Easy for us to say, but in reality, it may be critical. There are special circumstances and solutions to those ever-occurring exceptions:

Situation	Action
Page of any kind while in a patient's room.	Politely excuse yourself and answer the page.
During a case presentation.	Pager and cell phone set to vibrate. Better to give it to another person prior to your presentation. Quietly hand it to another person to answer for you.
Scrubbed in the operating room.	Ask circulator to answer your page.
As an observer at rounds.	Pager and cell phone set to vibrate. Sneak out. Call back briefly.
In the chief's office for counseling.	Give the pager or cell phone to a waiting colleague or to a secretary to screen the call.
While being berated by an attending or the page immediately.	Respectfully excuse yourself and respond to chief resident.

Chapter 7
Teaching and Learning

Experience is not what happens to you.
Experience is what you do with what happens
to you.

— Aldous Huxley

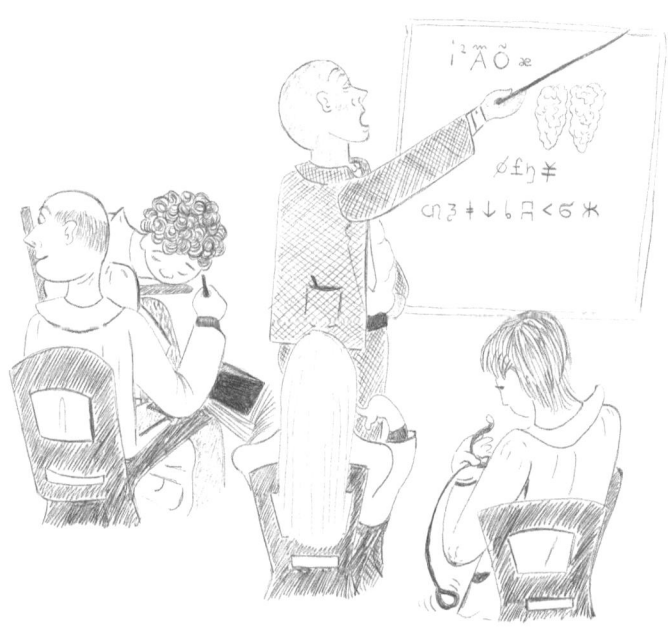

L.D. Florman, *The Portable Medical Mentor:*
Training Success, DOI 10.1007/978-3-319-09852-4_7,
© Springer International Publishing Switzerland 2015

7.1   Background

The whole purpose of your residency is to learn to function as an independent physician in whatever field you have chosen. Teaching and learning are an essential component to making a new doctor. If you are fortunate, you will have people around you who want to teach you all the essential components of your chosen specialty. If not, you will have to fend a little for yourself. This chapter is intended to do a few things:

1. Help you understand what you need to learn in your clinical years and in residency.
2. Help you locate resources to learn it.
3. Encourage you to develop "micro-lectures" to give to students and junior residents under your care.
4. Remind you of your role as a teacher to your patients.
5. Remind you of your role as a teacher to the rest of the healthcare profession.

A chapter on teaching and learning would not be complete without a word about our heritage. We certainly rest on the backs of giants in our profession. Take small opportunities to learn about the giants. Who is the father of modern anatomy? Andreas Vesalius in the sixteenth century wrote a six-volume treatise on anatomy. He did most of his dissections with the cadaver in the erect position so that the anatomy was more in a natural position. Who was Marie Cure? What did she die from? Who really first described Crohn's disease? No, it was not Crohn. Who were McBurney, La Forte, and the greats of medicine?

7.2   What You Need to Learn

Your most important job as a resident or fellow is not only to provide healthcare. It is to LEARN to provide healthcare. Your attendings and other residents are your teachers. It is their job to instruct you and your job to follow those instructions. Your program has a specific set of things it needs to teach you in order to be accredited by the ACGME. In fact, you will be graded on your ability to master each set of skills during your biannual evaluation that is now mandatory for all residents.

7.2.1 Surgery and the Surgical Specialties

For those of you in surgery and the surgical specialties, your operating room time can be argued to be the most important part of your education. Every case you go to is your opportunity to learn from it. DO NOT SHOW UP NOT KNOWING THE PATIENT, OR NOT HAVING READ ABOUT THE CASE. At least, not at first. If you have been working with the same three attendings in fellowship for 2 years, they will be more lenient. However, there is many a time where a resident has known or not known a critical piece of information that has led to an improvement of outcome for a patient. Show the attending you are knowledgeable about the operation, the patient, and can be counted on.

> *Attending: "Why can't we find the left URETER!?"*
> *Resident: "Remember her CT yesterday that said absent left kidney?"*
> *Attending: "Ah, glad you remembered!"*

Access surgery is a common database with links allowing you to read about virtually any operation at any time.

7.2.2 What Happens on the Floors and in the Clinics

This part of your education is arguably the more important, depending on who you talk to. You will be tested on your knowledge base daily. Not directly, but by patients and their conditions. Situations will test you. You have to be ready to answer. There are several key components to this.

One is to study your clinic patients. If possible, read about their conditions before you get to clinic. Read about what they have and what you can do about it. Know what your thoughts and options are before you see them. Most important, think ahead of time about how best to educate the patient about their disease, so that the treatment you recommend makes sense to them.

Another component is reading. There is no way around it—you WILL have to read a textbook covering your specialty at some point. Even if you just skim it and look at the helpful tables, you will need to pick a book, ANY BOOK, and read it.

7.3   Teaching

Teaching takes your reward to the next, and highest level, that of learning twice. While students and residents are still learners themselves, we expect them to serve as teachers and mentors to other medical students and fellow residents. We believe that teaching assists in solidification of one's own knowledge base and resident teaching helps attract medical students to the various fields of medicine.

Teaching a concept belies the underlying truth of your own familiarity with it. Teaching implies mastery. Think of the best grand rounds speaker you ever heard. The best ones were not standing there reciting their slides. They were instead instructing you on something they were experts in with years of experience and practical knowledge. This is the model you should endeavor to create as a teaching resident.

Remember that as a teacher, you have lots of tricks in your toolbox. If you don't know something then suggest—"Well, let's look that up." You look slick for being willing to help them find info, and you don't look dumb for not knowing something. Another trick, a favorite of many, is the prepared "micro-lecture." Think of things you know like the back of your hand that you could talk about without stopping for an hour or two. Then, distill that to its most basic 3 min. That thing needs to be given as a micro-lecture to the medical students on your service, every time you are around them.

You know a lot about gall bladder disease? Tell them, but remember what Wrigley said when everyone in America was buying his chewing gum after he virtually invented modern print advertising—"Tell 'em fast, tell 'em often." Make your learners repeat the information you deliver in some way (writing, orally) until they can tell you back what you told them. Then ask them the next day.

This sounds like a lot to ask someone who is averaging 80 h a week at work, is on call every third night, had a ton to read, and on and on. You are right; it is a lot to ask. It is, however, your duty. Also, you will find that by teaching the information, you will astound yourself at how much you sound like an attending when not hampered by the other conditions you constantly face.

7.3.1   Students as Learners

It is important as an instructor to remember your target audience. Medical students are for the most part eager, just as you were. They are also for the most part smart, just as you are. What most students have the hardest time with are the common questions that we ask them on the various rotations—the open-ended ones that we have been taught so well to ask our patients. Do not judge them harshly if they cannot answer swiftly in a grown-up way using real medical terms. They have not yet been taught to think medically and will have trouble thinking the way you do. Now here is the best part; it is YOUR job to help them think like you. That's the reason they are there.

Students are usually intimidated by residents and attendings in the medical disciplines. Try to soften this as much as you are able. They are paying a small fortune to spend time with you and learn, even if they are underfoot sometimes. As many things generally are, the best way to handle this directly is by simply saying, "Hey, welcome to the rotation. Don't be nervous. We want you to learn and have a good time. Watch out for this attending. No really, don't be nervous."

One of the best methods of teaching is letting students do as much as they are able to, safely. Students are always sick of waiting around and feeling aimless. If you can give a student a job, even if it seems menial to an intern, they feel like they contribute. Also, smaller tasks on your service allow the student to practice skills in interacting with patients, families, nurses, and other providers. Have students pull drains. Have students dictate notes. Have students write orders. The worse disservice you can do to a student is have them leave your service having learned some about the diseases you treat, but teaching them nothing about the practical everyday doctor things you take for granted. Engage them—make them work. THEY WILL LOVE YOU FOR IT. They will remember you. The faculty will remember you for it too.

7.3.2   Students Teaching Students

A great way to encourage and engage your students is to have them teach each other. You will have downtime during a day. It will come between cases, as you hang out on call, or any of the natural lulls between major movements as a resident. Have the students on the service prepare micro-lectures for each other. Grade the lectures. Give them feedback.

The other, KEY missing component that medical students crave is feedback.

Remember back to a time when people stopped grading you constantly—it was third year of medical school. That is when the constant influx of positive reinforcement is cut off in the lives of these young people. That can be pretty jarring. When there is no longer a teacher or professor consistently letting you know you are doing well by giving you a grade on an exam, paper, or what-have-you, it is very hard to perform any sort of self-evaluation. You can't know if the job you are doing is right because you don't know how to be a doctor.

This is MUCH worse on the wards. What makes a good student? Think about what your ideal student does—make it short. Tell the students at the beginning of the rotation, and hold them to that standard. And no, your ideal student cannot just leave you alone and study in the library all day. Though, sometimes you wish they would.

7.3.3   Students Teaching Residents (Yes They Can)

The notion may seem backwards at times. You will learn more from your students than you think. If there is something you want to know but don't have time to explore, have them look it up and tell you. You learn from them, and they get to feel useful. Win-win.

Beyond this, your interaction with students can inform you about your career choices. Like having students around and teaching all the time? Academics is for you. Just wish the students would go away so that you can do your work? Maybe that's a call to private practice. Remember, however, that even in private practice, you will be constantly teaching patients, families, nurses, and other doctors. You can never get away from teaching entirely as a doctor.

Remember, also, that students have experienced many of the specialties much more recently than you. They are your gateway to what is happening on rotations in the rest of the hospital. If you want to know the gut-check scoop about an attending? Ask the student who has rotated with them before. The students will know what has been going on with the other services, if they are savvy. They can also tell you what is old news in the medical world according to people you don't interact with — "Well, we really don't check that lab any more according to what Dr. Smith said when I was on Rheumatology last month." Leverage this to the best of your ability.

7.3.4   Residents Teaching Residents

Part of your job will be showing other residents the ropes of how to function as a specialist. You are modeling a role for them on a daily basis. What you do as a senior resident, the juniors will believe to be ok. Teach them how to trust and respect the support staff, by showing them how.

There will be several procedures that you have to teach residents how to do. Make sure that you are comfortable performing it as well as teaching it. Practice it mentally. Practice your teaching mentally quickly before you begin. Make sure that the procedure is level and ability appropriate. Again, ask them to repeat the essential steps when you are done.

7.3.5   Everybody Teaching Hospital Personnel

The nurses and personnel you come into contact with may not have the most current or correct medical information. You will be called on to teach them, virtually every day. This is a great way to get RNs up to speed, but it also builds your rapport with the nurses who will one day save you from making a significant mistake.

Your teaching for this crowd can take many forms. A simple comment about a particular situation is usually sufficient to educate an individual nurse. It is a good idea, though, to think about giving grand rounds for nurses or other formal lectures. Nurses are very connected throughout your community and speak freely. They can be an excellent source of referrals.

Also, don't be so quick to judge—the nurses have a lot to teach you as well. Among the best things you can do as a junior resident is ask the nurse how to handle a situation you are unfamiliar with. Often, the nurse will educate you on the way to deal with standard patient issues that come up all the time. A favorite tactic is to ask nurses, "What else should we be doing? What else to you need to take good care of my patient?"

7.3.6   Everybody Teaching Patients and Families

This role is among your most important as a doctor. You will be called upon daily to explain in layman's terms what exactly is going on with a patient. Your job is to tell the truth in a way that the patient will understand. Your goal is to have them be able to articulate their predicament to their family and friends—that way you know they truly understand.

Employ all the methods of a great teacher. Use anatomic models (often free from drug companies). Use illustrations — several better attendings go so far as to practice drawing the illustrations they will make for patients as a means of explanation.

Remember — a teacher can be anyone. We are all learning all the time. You should learn something new in medicine every day. If you don't, you aren't really practicing, you're just showing up.

Chapter 8
Surgery Suite Etiquette

"Small opportunities are often the beginning of great enterprises."

—Demosthenes

8.1 Background

Demosthenes was a powerful orator of ancient Greece who captivated his audience despite a speech impediment. He taught himself to speak distinctly by talking with pebbles in his mouth. To strengthen his voice, he spoke over the roar of the waves at the seashore. Demosthenes had a "great enterprise" but a "small opportunity" to improve his speech impediment and achieve success. One great enterprise in medicine is to improve the working relationships that surround you so that those relationships can run more effectively and grow stronger. In this chapter, we will discuss scheduling procedures, preoperative activities, conduct in the operating room, and postoperative activities.

This chapter is meant for the medical student about to undertake his rotation on the surgical services, and no less to the resident and fellow in surgery. Some attending surgeons would do well to study this chapter. Students will not have the opportunity to take a leadership role in most of the items discussed below. They can be vigilant observers, learning

L.D. Florman, *The Portable Medical Mentor: Training Success*, DOI 10.1007/978-3-319-09852-4_8,
© Springer International Publishing Switzerland 2015

how a fine-tuned machine such as the operating room environment could or should work.

Surgery is a preemptive specialty, demanding innovation, organization, and the ability to rapidly adapt one's thinking methods. These are all learned functions. They do not come naturally; however, once observed correctly, they will simply become the way of life for the student and resident in surgery.

8.2   Scheduling

The operating room can be your "kingdom," but you are the ruler of this domain only as long as your reputation holds up. So, why not protect and enhance your domain and your reputation before you are placed into a position of authority? As the "crown prince," your reputation will be judged as to how you behave in the operating suite and it all starts with scheduling. Sometimes scheduling is a function completed for you by others; however, quite often, you must schedule the procedure yourself. Whether the patients are from the clinic or private office, have elective or emergency surgeries, make every effort to schedule the procedure yourself. Do not assign this important function to a nurse or secretary. The advantages are enormous. Note: Generally, only chief residents, fellows, and attending may schedule cases in the operating suite.

Start Time. You have the advantage of negotiating the starting time of the procedure if you schedule it yourself. The scheduler can hear from your own mouth the exact nature of the procedure (i.e., the urgency, the lack of urgency, the type, and quality of the personnel to place in the room), and by knowing you can better determine how long the procedure will really take. You must realize that there are fast surgeons and there are ones who are not so fast. There are those of us who can be trusted to estimate time rather accurately, and there are those who will overestimate, or usually underestimate times in an effort to inflate their own egos, or will just not know. If you (or your attending) are particularly slow, then honestly inform the scheduler that you will need more time to perform the procedure. Remember, you may fool the scheduler the first time, but not the second time. The second time the scheduler will remember you, and could set your start time to begin around 2:45 a.m. to merely excise a small skin lesion.

Do not upset the scheduler or supervisory operating staff. Sometimes it is difficult to control oneself when people are not cooperating as you wish. Remember, these people have been working long before you came, and will continue long after you leave. They have the ear of the attendings and never mind telling them how evil you were towards them. That will register adversely with your attending and the chief.

Equipment and Supplies. By scheduling the procedure yourself, you have an opportunity to inform the scheduler precisely what equipment and supplies you will require. There is nothing wrong with being very specific. Have everything you need in the room before you start, so that you do not have to run the circulator ragged searching for, let's say, a 6-0 nylon on a P-1 needle.

Personnel. You may have the opportunity to request specific personnel. This is particularly desirable if you can arrange it, but be careful not to offend others.

Working Relationships. Take advantage of the opportunity to develop a working relationship with the scheduler or scheduling department. There will always be special times when you need a really big favor. You may need to schedule a case a bit earlier in order to make your wedding anniversary an "event" instead of a "memory." Be polite, respectful, and honest. Try it; you will be pleased with the results.

Drawbacks. One of the drawbacks of scheduling procedures yourself is that you will have nobody to blame but yourself when things don't go precisely as you planned.

Suggestions:

Schedule early.
Schedule honestly.

Identify yourself by name and service.

Schedule all of the various parts of the operation.

Make sure that the scheduler knows the severity of the case.

Make sure that the scheduler knows the proposed duration of the case.

Make sure that the scheduler knows of any special equipment needs.

Place your attending's name first.

Be polite, succinct, and respectful.

Say "thank you" before you hang up.

8.3   Preoperative Activities

Your efforts in the preoperative period will be noted by your attendings and the nursing staff. This is certainly the most important aspect of surgery for the junior house staff member, as your superiors count on your thoroughness. This period begins when the condition of the patient is discerned and ends with the surgical intervention. It is your job to be up to date on all aspects of your patient's care and to keep your superiors notified of any changes. Expect calls from superiors at the most inconvenient times and be prepared to answer some very specific questions. One faulty step at times like this will require ten positive ones to correct it.

Assume Responsibility. Many of these suggestions may not be your direct responsibility, but if not carried out properly, you are the one who will pay the price. Once these routines are established, you will become very efficient at accomplishing them. In fact, you may make a real difference from time to time.

Notes and Orders. Review progress notes and nursing notes at least twice a day. If a consultant has been asked to examine the patient, continuously watch for his note and any follow-up notes. Review the orders at least twice a day. Others may have written orders for tests, or studies, and you MUST know the results.

Reports. Watch closely for addendums to X-ray results and pathology reports. These can be critical in the care of your patient.

Wounds. If a wound is involved, make sure that you examine it daily as well as just prior to surgery.

Communicate. Remind and brief the nursing staff of the impending surgery. If possible, discuss the surgery with the patient. If this has already been done by your superior, you should still ask the patient whether he has any questions. Certainly do not refute anything that any staff has told your patient without first checking with that staff person. Get a little personal with the patient. Ask the patient if there is anything that you can do to be of help. Discuss the surgery with the family if appropriate, but be ever cognizant of HIPAA rules. Remember, this is a particularly stressful time for the patient and the family.

Consent. Double check that the patient has informed consent. Again, be careful that you do not refute or confuse anything that your superiors may have told the patient. Check that the "consent for surgery" has been properly signed and witnessed. Many surgeries have been canceled in the operating room because of an improperly executed consent.

Document. Document in the progress notes that you obtained consent and whether there were any family members present. If necessary, dictate a short note outlining that you spoke to the patient about risks and benefits, and that everyone had an opportunity to ask questions.

This is a good time to remember to mark the patient. It is a JCAOH (Joint Commission on Accreditation of Hospitals) rule that all operative sites must be marked before the patient comes to the operating room. This simple but necessary procedure has drastically reduced the number of wrong-sided surgeries.

Prepare. If you have not already done so, review the nature of the patient's condition, the anatomy, and the finer points of the proposed surgery. Whether you are junior or senior, be sure that you are up to date on the most current readings. Fortuitous occurrences have a way of happening. If you are the first-year resident and the senior resident has to attend an emergency, you may be next in line to do the case with the attending.

BE PREPARED.
KNOW THE ANATOMY.

8.4   Operating Room Conduct

You will be judged by your peers, your superiors, your attendings, the operating personnel, and your patients, by your actions in the operating room. Bad actions will be noted and discussed ad nauseam by all. It is your reputation, and you should protect it with your every effort. Your good actions will be quietly noted but loudly passed on to others. You will gain the admiration or scorn by those that surround you and those at a distance. Of course, this applies to everything you do in your training, but in the operating suite those bad and good actions are accentuated. The good actions will gain you praise from all, thus reinforcing your frail ego.

You will note your fellow house staffers do many of the items we are going to talk about, and you will be impressed with them. It should be your desire to do all of the things that we suggest. We can teach you technique, but that is not our mission. The technique will come with experience and a lot of extracurricular practice.

Prepare. Study the disease and the anatomy before entering the operating room suite. Be the "world expert." Read at least two recent articles in the literature and be ready to discuss them in the doctor's lounge, in the hallways, and over the operating table. Sometimes you will not have the opportunity to show what you know. Other times you will find the opportune time to interject your new knowledge. Your superiors will be pleased to tell their friends and colleagues about the great resident who works with them and who is always prepared.

Study the operation long before entering the operating room. You should not be in the operating room without a thorough knowledge of the surgical anatomy and the technical operation.

Reports. It is essential to have all lab reports and original X-rays in the operating room. Today, most of these items are in the computer system and can be easily transmitted directly into the operating room. This is your job. This is not the time to be fumbling for the correct X-rays.

Time. <u>Always</u> be in the operating suite early. Visit the patient in the holding area. Start times must be adhered to. In most, if not all hospitals, the start time is the "cut time." Do everything in your power to have that patient in the room in a timely fashion. Beg the nurses. Entice the anesthesiologist. Prod your attending. Remember, if your case is late in finishing, the case to follow will also be late. This is not the way to win friends. Holdups seem to cascade, and delays become additive. You can make sure that your patient is sent for from the hospital room early enough. Even though it may not be your job, you will look very good if you can speed up the process.

Be Helpful. Ask the circulator and scrub nurse what you can do to help. When they help, you should remember to say "thank you."

Music in the Operating Room. Gently demand that the room be as quiet as possible. One word about music in the operating room: If you have it, make it subdued. If the attending who is responsible for you in the operating room does not like music, then do not bring it into the room. If anybody in the room objects to the music, then turn it off. If the patient is awake, make the music calming, not rock and roll.

Stay Put. Once the patient is in the operating room, never leave until it is time to wash your hands. Stay with your patient. Talk to him. Touch him. Comfort him. This is an extremely difficult and stressful time for every patient, regardless of his bravado. Problems occur during induction of anesthesia. Another pair of expert hands may be necessary. Your calm and reassuring demeanor is mandatory. Gently demand that the room be as quiet as possible. No extraneous conversation. The center of conversation must be the patient at all times. The patient expects it and does not want to hear about the great movie nurse Smith saw last night.

Be careful what you and others say in the operating during general anesthesia. We have all heard stories about the supposedly anesthetized patient who heard every derogatory word the surgeon said during her operation.

Consider this experience as a lesson learned:

A middle-aged African/American woman was prone on the operating table being submitted to spine surgery. The surgeons were discussing last night's Passover meal. The surgery went well, except that the surgeons were operating on the wrong two disks. The next morning during routine rounds the surgeons asked the patient if everything was going well. She stated that she was not at all happy as she heard the entire conversation that took place during her surgery, that she was wide awake during the entire procedure, but couldn't move, and that she didn't like being called a "fat pig." When challenged by the surgeons, saying that was impossible, she said "then how do I now know the recipe for matza-ball soup?" Everybody was sued, including the surgeons, the nurses, the hospital, the anesthesiologists, and the manufacturer of the anesthesia equipment. Everybody lost and paid money.

Skin Prep. Somebody (you) must be present for the entire skin prep, closely observing for any break in sterile procedure. Just because a senior or a very experienced nurse does the prep, this does not mean that it is correct.

Assume Responsibility. As you gain more responsibilities, there are several things that you can do to make surgery run smoother. Write down a list of your needed equipment and supplies and give it to the circulator before the patient enters the operating room. Notify the staff of the patient's special needs so that they can comport themselves accordingly.

Show the scrub nurse what instruments you believe should be on the Mayo stand and what instruments certainly will not be used. Tell the staff the "order" of the operation.

Scrubbing. Scrub your hands as you would want your surgeon to do for your operation. Proper etiquette dictates that if you are scrubbing with an attending, you should finish when he is finished. Attempt to scrub, gown, and glove, and help the scrub nurse drape the patient before your superiors enter the room.

Time-Out. In 2004 the Joint commission for Accreditation of Hospitals approved and mandated the "Universal Protocol for Preventing Wrong Site, Wrong Procedure and Wrong Person Surgery." These rules apply to all accredited hospitals and ambulatory care and office-based surgery facilities. This protocol involves three steps:

1. Conduct a pre-procedure verification process.
2. Mark the procedure site.
3. Perform a time-out in the operating room.
   This a formal, dedicated time before the operation begins. Everybody in the operating room plays a part.

   - The patient is positively identified.
   - The operation is identified.
   - The site of surgery is identified.
   - Allergies.
   - Medications.

   Document the completion of the time-out.

While you are waiting around, scrubbed and ready to operate, check the Mayo stand with all the instruments the scrub nurse has accumulated. Go through the operation in your mind. See if there are any instruments not present. Better to have too many instruments than not enough. Better to have too many sutures in the room than to have the circulator run around for them.

Assisting or Starting. If you are prepared in your knowledge of the technique and the anatomy, now is the correct time to ask your attending in a polite, humble way: "May I start"? He may very well respond affirmatively and permit you to do the entire operation, or at least until you stumble.

Be Assertive. Depending on what your role is to be at the table (i.e.. surgeon, first assistant, second assistant … fifth assistant), you may assume that physical position. Actually, why not presume that by some twist of faith the boss is going to give you the case. So, why not just assume the position of the surgeon, and see what transpires. Whether or not you are given the case, it demonstrates to others that because of your preparation, you are willing and able to assume the title of "surgeon." Even if this bold technique fails, you will stand a good chance of being the first assistant. If applied correctly, the above suggestion will show others that you are definitely willing, able, knowledgeable, and certainly assertive, which are all good traits for a young aspiring surgeon.

There is nothing wrong with taking preemptive roles. If he is sewing, take a needle holder with suture and ask if you can sew also. Don't ask, and then take the needle holder. Take the needle holder, and then ask. If there is a bleeder that is staring at you, stop it. If you can expose something with a retractor, then move the retractor or get another one.

Make every attempt to anticipate the next three moves of the surgeon, the next instrument needed, the next suture needed, the type of bandage that will be used, and the situation of the next patient for the operating room. In other words, be the very best first assistant.

Idiosyncrasies. Learn by experience the idiosyncrasies of each surgeon you work with. At the end of each procedure make a note in your little black book (see Chap. 3) about his likes and dislikes and refer to these notes before the next case. The note might include what kind of suture he likes, how many throws in his knots, the kind of dressing, the technique, the music in the operating room, his favorite discussion subject, etc. Check with the residents who preceded you on the service for their advice.

Finishing Up. The operation is not finished until the patient is in the recovery room. You place the bandage as instructed. You stay with the patient. You help lift the patient on to the recovery stretcher. You help wheel the patient to the recovery area. You give any special instructions to the recovery personnel.

Thank You. When leaving the operating room, sincerely thank each person individually. Shake the hand of the anesthetist. Thank the nurse for handing you the instruments, and your circulator for running to the basement for a cotton ball. Do not miss anybody. Do it even if you were holding the fifth retractor and did not get any blood on your gloves. Some of them will look at you hesitatingly. All of them will remember you and the small gesture of appreciation you gave them. It goes a very long way. Do this for the rest of your career.

8.5   Postoperative Activities

If you are given the responsibility of writing the post-op note and orders, you better check with the surgeon for the exact title of the operation. This is very important for reimbursement and legal reasons. Make sure that the recovery room personnel are comfortable with the written post-op orders and the patient's overall condition. You should frequently check with the recovery room to determine when the patient is transferred to the floor.

Although it may not be your job, you can certainly assure yourself that someone has spoken to the patient's family. It is a good practice to go to the waiting room with your attending or superior. The attending will appreciate the entourage, and you will learn the techniques of speaking to families, and how not to speak to families.

Chapter 9
The Clinics

*"Give what you have. To someone, it may be
better than you dare think."*

— Henry Wadsworth Longfellow

9.1   Institutional Clinics

The performance of each institutional clinic will differ by title
and by rules. In general, however, there are similarities,
regardless of institution, department, specialty, state, or local
rules. For instance, clinic patients should be treated no differently from your private patients, whether they were paying
you for your advice and services, or not. On the other hand,
just as in private practice, you will equally encounter difficult
individuals (see Chap. 11) or have unusual problems in the
clinics. All patients must receive the best of care, even if you
do not like the patient. With the help of your attending physician, this should not be a problem. Remember, you are in
training to be a physician, but the patient is not practicing to
be ill. They are counting on you to provide them the care that
they need.

   An attending physician will be in charge of the clinic. Very
often, he will be present during most, if not all, of your time.
Every patient must be discussed with him. By experience, he
is equipped to not only teach you, but also "scope out" the

L.D. Florman, *The Portable Medical Mentor:*   53
Training Success, DOI 10.1007/978-3-319-09852-4_9,
© Springer International Publishing Switzerland 2015

occasional "red herring." Also, he is morally, ethically, and legally responsible for what occurs in your clinic. Be sure to tell him of your successes in treatment as well as your failures, and certainly all complications, no matter how trivial they may appear.

Since these are, in essence, your private patients, you must be on time for your clinic, be appropriately dressed, and behave correctly. Appear and act as the doctor you would want caring for a member of your family. The nursing staff is very busy during clinic hours. Try not to make too many demands of them at this time. Specifically, if there is anything that you can do, then do it yourself.

Here are specific points that are worth noting while you are in the clinics:

1. Entering the examining room:

   • Knock lightly on the examining room door before entering. You should not wait for an invitation to enter.
   • Introduce yourself by title and last name. Never with your first name. Greet your patient by title and last name. Children may be greeted by their first name.
   • Most patients will address you as doctor.
   • Be careful to know the rules for unescorted minors. The nurse should be familiar with the local rules. If not, consult with your attending.
   • Never enter an examining room with a female patient unless accompanied by a female nurse or the reverse order for female physicians. This rule can be altered if a family member, close friend, significant other, or caregiver is present. Having these individuals in the examining room also takes some pressure off the patient to explain the reason for the visit, and allows another set of ears to listen to the doctor's comments and instructions.
   • Be pleasant, interested, considerate, respectful, professional, and thorough.

2. Communicating with patients:

   • Always speak plain English to patients. They do not understand medical terms, slang, abbreviations, or initials.

Even if they are very sophisticated, they will want to hear "plain English" when it comes to their health.

- If there is a language barrier, then a translator should be present.
- There is nothing wrong with a little familiarity.
- With certain individuals a bit of humor is often welcome.

3. Examining referred patients:

- When seeing a patient in consultation, who is referred from another physician or clinic, an attempt should be made to call that physician with your report. The minimum response should be to send him a copy of your history and physical examination and your plan for the future care of the patient. The immediate response can just be a telephone call. These items take a little longer to perform, but are always appreciated by the referring doctor. They will also generate more respect for you, your clinic, and your service, as well as more referrals.
- A word about "dumps":
  A "dump" might be considered a patient who is thrown upon you by another physician or clinic, for the purpose of ridding oneself of that patient. In reality, there is no such thing as a "dump." Each patient who is seen in your clinic deserves independent and appropriate care. A bad referral does not reflect on the patient as much as it does on the referring doctor. Also, this occurrence provides you with the opportunity to be a star, a hero, and sometimes to make a diagnosis and/or a treatment that others have missed.

4. Observing the patient:

- Be ever vigil of drug abuse in your patients.
- Watch for child abuse.
- Watch for elder abuse.
- Observe carefully the demeanor of the caregivers.

5. Follow up with the patient:

- If you promise to call a patient with any information, then you must call them at the appointed time. Put it in your "little black book" along with the phone number.
- Do not allow the nursing staff to make your calls for you.
- Do not communicate with patients by e-mail. You cannot be sure that they received the message.
- Remember, when calling a patient; speak to no one except the patient or the person who is legally responsible (HIPAA).
- You must follow up with patient on all salient lab reports. Biopsy reports must be relayed to the patient as soon as they are available.

6. Exiting the examining room:

- Never permanently discharge a patient from your clinic until his condition is completely resolved or he has been appropriately referred to another healthcare provider. Once this has occurred, write in the chart the precise disposition of the patient and "return prn."
- Always offer the patient the ability to return to the clinic or to call you directly in case of any problem with their condition.

7. Writing in the patient's chart:

- Make sure that a patient's chart does not disappear into the system before you are able to write in it.
- Write all notes or complete the Electronic Medical Record immediately following the visit.
- Request that your attending sign all charts contemporaneously.
- Do not remove charts from the clinic.
- With the advent of the Electronic Medical Record, institutional compliance with the timeliness of reports has become easier. The institution is keeping track of you and will record and notify you and your superiors of any lacks in compliance.

8. <u>Ending each clinic:</u>

- At the end of each clinic, look at each name on the clinic list, making sure that nothing has been missed. Make sure that all aspects of the electronic medical record have been adhered to.
- Check the "no-shows" at the end of every clinic and take appropriate action when necessary. If the nursing staff handles no-shows, then frequently check with the nursing staff. No-shows can get you into a lot of trouble.
- Any lab or imaging studies that are scheduled must be followed up by you in a very timely fashion. Write down the type of test in your "little black book," along with the phone number so that you can call the patient with the results.
- If you are the more senior resident at the clinic, you must be informed about every patient that your juniors examine, before the patient leaves the clinic.

9.2   The Private Office

There are at least three scenarios in which you might find yourself in an attending's private office. First, an attending surgeon may offer you the opportunity to spend time with him in his private practice. If he does, consider it an honor that he thinks so much of you that he is allowing you to not only be introduced to his private patients, but also see how his office functions and observe a portion of his personal life. Second, you may have a mandatory rotation in the private office. This should be considered a mandatory opportunity. Third, in a pinch, your attending may ask you to work in his private office to perform a small function such as to remove sutures, inspect a wound, or even to deliver lunch. Regardless of the reason, you must grasp these opportunities and treat them respectfully and gleefully, since the transition from the clinic to the private office is the beginning of your transition into the real world of private practice. Dress and groom immaculately. Be gracious, humorous, courteous, and curious to the private office staff. Do not question the attending in front of his patient. In the examining room, stand straight with your hands out of your pockets, and do not lean against the wall or read your text messages.

These visits to the private office could ultimately become a type of interview for a job or possibly the beginning of a dialogue for a partnership. Do not take lightly the importance of the office staff and their uncanny ability to sway their bosses' opinion about everything from the brand of paper towels to buy to the kind of doctor they would want to have in <u>their</u> office.

9.3   Clinic vs. Private Office

In most medical institutions in the country there is a very definite distinction between "clinic" and "private office." "Clinic" most often denotes a medical facility. "Office" or "private office" is the place where a faculty member or private practitioner sees patients. These patients may be clinic type patients or private patients. Historically, and today, there is often a feeling that clinic patients are indigent and cannot afford to be seen in the private office. Of course, that is not always the case.

Be a little sensitive when using the words. Go along with the prevailing vernacular of the attending physicians in the clinics and offices in which you participate.

Chapter 10
Rounds

"If you get all the facts, your judgment could be right; if you don't get all the facts, it can't be right."

—Bernard M. Baruch

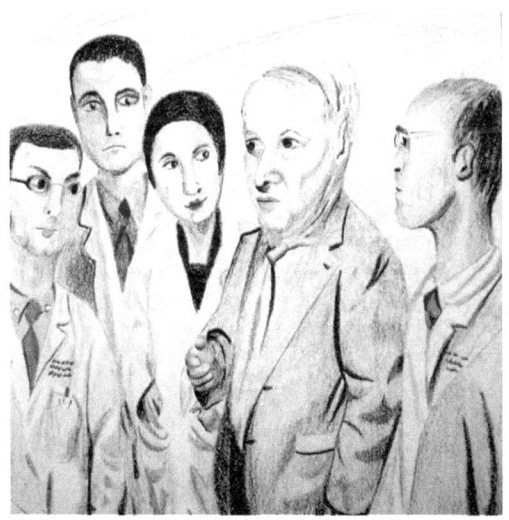

Fig. 10.1. Patient rounds

L.D. Florman, *The Portable Medical Mentor:*
Training Success, DOI 10.1007/978-3-319-09852-4_10,
© Springer International Publishing Switzerland 2015

10.1 General

Every institution has its own definition of, and vocabulary for, rounds. For the purposes of this publication, we will define rounds as the time when you regularly see patients in the hospital. Every patient must be seen by the resident (not just the student) at least once a day, and the resident (not the student) must write a note in the patient's chart. Most patients will be seen more than once a day. The first rounds of the day should occur prior to scheduled surgery, lectures, conferences, and meetings. This will indeed assure you of having to wake very early. It will also assure you that the patient will not be distracted by breakfast or that too many relatives or friends will be present.

Proper writing in the patient's chart or Electronic Medical Record will be covered elsewhere (see Chaps. 12 and 26). What follows are just a few points about rounds that must become automatic forever more:

• Write patient notes immediately following the visit.
• Sign the chart, date it, and write down the time.
• Verbally tell the nurse of all orders in addition to writing them in the patient's chart.
• Do not enter a female patient's room without a female nurse, or family member.
• Politely request that all extraneous visitors leave the patient's room, with the exception of one or two family members, if appropriate.
• Following rounds, seek out any family members, if appropriate.
• When with others on rounds:

  – Speak clearly and loud enough for everyone in your group to hear.
  – Use note cards.
  – Do not memorize a script; it sounds bad.
  – If you stumble, continue with a smile. Do not apologize for mispronounced words; attempt only once to correct it.

– Try to anticipate all of the questions that you could be asked, and build the answers into your presentation. Do not guess at an answer. Do not make excuses for omissions in diagnoses or treatments. Never lie. Do not blame anybody for anything.

A few scenarios:

10.2   Rounds by Yourself

- If appropriate, introduce yourself, or remind the patient who you are.
- Dress appropriately (tie, pressed pants, pants and blouse, dress, clean white lab coat). (Flormanism: Dress like your mother would like to see you in her hospital room.)
- Apologize if you wake the patient.
- Arrange to have a female nurse with you if the patient is female (or the reverse in case of a female physician).
- If dressing changes are needed, the supplies should already be in the room, having been ordered by you the day before, so as not to waste time. Always think ahead.
- When you leave the room, assure the patient if and when you will return.

10.3   Rounds with Residents and/or Students

- If anyone is not dressed appropriately, send them to correct the problem(s).
- It is a good idea to have a more junior person go on rounds before you and undress the wound, if appropriate. If you are the more junior person, then offer to go ahead.
- Do not whisper to others in hopes that the patient will not hear.
- Use medical language judiciously. Try not to use medical talk to the students, residents, and nurses in the room.
- Since anything that is said in the room with a negative connotation may be misunderstood by the patient, do not use

innuendos, jargon, double entendres, or initials. Patients tend to perceive your every word in a very literal fashion.
- Be sure that a fresh dressing is placed immediately. If the nurse is to do this, then ask the student or junior resident to check to see whether it was done.
- Be aware of sensitive issues concerning the patient, such as psychiatric problems, addictions, or family matters.

10.4   Rounds with Attendings

- Students: This is a large opportunity. Be noticeable. Stand in the front, near the presenter, or near the attending. Do not stand in the back with all your fellow students. You will not be noticed.
- Dress appropriately (tie, pants and blouse, dress, clean white lab coat). Make sure that everyone is appropriately dressed.
- Prior to rounds, the patient's dressings should be removed, wounds exposed, and lightly covered.
- Any relevant imaging studies or lab and pathology results should be available. Use note cards as needed.
- If your attending does not know the details of the patient, then make a formal presentation. If your attending is current on this patient, then only update him on the relevant changes.
- Do not permit any one to argue with or undermine the authority of the attending while in the patient's room.
- Nudge any discussion out of the room and into the hall, allowing everyone an opportunity to ask questions and make comments. This also tends to decrease anxiety in the patient.

10.5   Rounds with the Chief

- Students: This is the largest opportunity. Be noticeable. Stand in the front, near the presenter, or near the attending. Do not stand in the back with all of your fellow students. You will not be noticed.

- Dress appropriately, but do not necessarily dress like him. Wear a clean white coat and look fresh. No scrubs, unless the boss is wearing them. Anyone who is not appropriately dressed should be sent away. This will only happen one time.
- If this is a spur-of-the-moment visit, then someone should call ahead and have the nurse or your junior resident undress the wound, ask the family members to leave the room, turn off the TV, and prepare the patient about what to expect when making rounds with the boss. If you are the junior, then do this yourself. Make your senior look good. He'll remember you.
- Any description of the patient should be made on the way to the room, not inside the room.
- Be very brief, very succinct, and very clear.
- Always end your presentation with a plan for treatment.

10.6   Weekly Rounds

Each training program will approach weekly rounds differently. These are often held at the bedside, in an auditorium, or a conference room, and involve many people (the chief, attendings, residents, fellows, specialties, students, nursing, ancillary personnel), perhaps as many as 30–50. This is your chance to excel or crash. **BE PREPARED**.

10.6.1   If You Are the Presenter of Weekly Rounds

- Wear a clean shirt, tie, and crisp white lab coat. Bring one pen, one flashlight (optional), no papers hanging out of your pockets. Place the stethoscope in your pocket (or absent), not around your neck.
- Shined shoes.
- Get there early.
- Be very familiar with the patient's entire chart.
- Be familiar with what is not in the chart (social history).

– Be familiar with the patient's hospital course.
– Know all lab values of the patient.
– Have imaging films and reports available.
– Politely ask family members and others to wait in the waiting room.
– Turn off the patient's TV.
– Make a simple but detailed, computer-generated, bold-typed summary of the history, hospital course, operations, and timeline.
– Stand straight, hands out of the pockets, and maintain good eye contact with everyone in attendance.
– Address the crowd individually and as a group.
– No leaning against the wall. No looking at the floor or ceiling. Do not use too many abbreviations or initials. Keep your hands away from your face and mouth.
– Don't be cute.
– Speak very clearly; do not waste time with extraneous facts.

10.6.2   If You Are a Helper at Weekly Rounds (Student or Junior Resident)

– Make the presenter's life easier during this really anxiety-laden period of time. He will do the same for you.
– Do his computer work, fetch, and set up the X-rays, turn off the TV, undress the wound, and make it look pretty.
– Tell the patient what is about to happen and why.
– Support your senior in any way that you can. Physically and emotionally stand beside him.

10.6.3   If You Are a Listener at Weekly Rounds

– Comply with the same dress code.
– Be noticeable.
– No secondary conversations.
– No chewing gum.
– Do not hesitate to ask questions. Avoid comments, unless addressed by an attending. **Look interested**.

10.7   Grand Rounds

Grand rounds are often held in an auditorium with many in attendance. In times gone by, these conferences would center on the presentation of a particular patient, followed by an in-depth presentation and discussion of the disease and treatment with which the patient presented. Now, these grand rounds usually are didactic sessions on a particular subject. They are often relegated to local or visiting experts. Not infrequently, a senior resident will be asked to present. Needless to say, this is a very important hour for a resident, taking much time for preparation and thought. Every point reviewed in this chapter should be adhered to.

Grand rounds are often attended by all of the faculty as well as practitioners outside of the institution. This makes the conference the "pride" of the department, proudly showing the best of their residents and the active participation of the community surgeons.

10.8   Teach, Teaching, and Teachers

This chapter on rounds is a good place to remind students, interns, and residents that teaching and learning is the primary goal of your education, and that the instillation of practical knowledge and technical skills is a learned function, taught by those who learned it just as you are learning from others. Regardless of your level of training, you are now the teacher and the student. You will be delighted to discover that teaching others is also an education for the teacher, a sort of learning twice. It is your privilege and duty to pass along your growing knowledge. One's education in medicine demands the direct interactions between teacher and student, where both teacher and student depend on each other for their education.

It has been estimated that 40–50 % of a resident's training is due to the efforts of fellow house staff (Brown, Robert S., "Staff Attitudes toward Teachings." *Journal of Medical*

Education 45: 156–158, 1970); therefore, it is essential that interns and residents at all levels become good teachers. It is unfortunate that very little is taught to medical students, interns, and residents on the subject and art of teaching. There are techniques to teaching effectively in a superb little book (Thomas L. Schwenk, M.D., Neal Whitman, Ed.D., *Residents as Teachers: A Guide to Educational Practice*, 1993, University of Utah School of Medicine) that will help you not only be the best teacher that you can be, but also a better learner.

10.9   Note

Remember, medical knowledge is not proprietary. It is meant to be graciously shared. There is no need for residents and interns in surgery to compete. Everybody who performs well performs well for the group. There are no bell-shaped curves for student, intern, and resident prowess. You are judged on what you do and how well your group does. Do not compete with or against your colleagues. Have a burning desire that they all will do well. It will make you look good to make them look good.

Chapter 11
The Difficult

"Kind words can be short and easy to speak, but their echoes are truly endless."

—Mother Teresa

Effectively dealing with the difficult person (i.e., patient, family member, colleague, attending, consultant, hospital personnel) can almost be considered an art form, but this type of expertise may not be taught as an exacting science, nor does it come naturally to most young doctors, or to many older doctors. It is learned from experience, maturity, and compassion. And, this knowledge must come very quickly, as the difficult person can enter your life when you least expect it and have a profound effect on you and the individual as well. The one saving grace about the difficult person is that you can often predict the difficulty before it occurs, so you should have time to figure out what to do prior to any misunderstanding or, better yet, prevent it from occurring in the first place.

11.1 The Difficult Patient

First, do not prejudge your patient. You may listen to others' evaluation of the patient, but it is far better to interact with him or her as though you are going to have an exemplary

L.D. Florman, *The Portable Medical Mentor:*
Training Success, DOI 10.1007/978-3-319-09852-4_11,
© Springer International Publishing Switzerland 2015

doctor/patient relationship from the start. If things go downhill from there, then you must critically evaluate the possible causes.

Was it you? Ask yourself these questions: Was your greeting incorrect? Were you not dressed and groomed appropriately? Did you not show appropriate respect? Were you too casual, too arrogant? Were you too "medical" and not "down-to-earth?" Could they read in your eyes and in your body movements that you might have lacked compassion, didn't understand the problem, didn't care, were in a hurry, or were preoccupied? Could they see by your questions and/or your examination that you did not have the expertise necessary to help them?

Remember, there is nothing more important to patients than their medical condition and their desire to return to health. This is what all patients think about; this is all they want you to think about. Most patients are quite nervous when the doctor visits. They forget to mention certain things, and they forget to ask important questions. It is up to you to draw questions and answers out of them and to be sure that the patient is comfortable with and understands what you are telling them. Go slowly. Be thorough. Be compassionate. Be respectful.

Was it them? Were they distracted by their condition, pain, not feeling well, and medications? Did something happen? A problem with another doctor? A problem with the nursing staff? A problem with family or at home? A problem with work? Angry at the world because they are sick? Angry that they are not sick? Lost hope? Do they have a psychiatric problem?

This is when all of your skills of understanding and patience come into play. These difficult patients must be converted into normal patients as expeditiously as possible. If there is a correctible issue (and there almost always is), then you must take the time and expend the energy to understand it, have the perseverance to investigate it, and have the compassion to make it right. Always remember that the patient is the real endpoint of your education and training. Do not fail the patient.

There is nothing wrong with involving others in assisting you with these problems. Psychiatrists, social workers, and nursing supervisors are most valuable in these situations and should be used liberally. It will come to pass that, even through your best efforts, you may not succeed in getting through to the difficult patient. There may come a time when you will find it necessary to request assistance from a senior doctor, even perhaps the chief. Do not wait too long to do this, as the condition will grow worse rapidly.

Be sure to write the details of each encounter in the patient's chart. It is important to use exact quotations, and these should be documented with quotation marks.

11.2   The Difficult Family Member

First, be sure that you are dealing with a true family member or a person who is legally responsible for the patient. Do not forget HIPAA (Chap. 24). When you are talking to a group of family members, you must identify each one in the group, and you must be sure that each person is comfortable with you speaking to the group. Keep in mind that the motivations of family members can be widely varied.

Difficult family members can often be more challenging to handle than difficult patients. The same rules of conduct apply to them as to patients. Be respectful, understanding, and compassionate. Take as much time as needed to explain the patient's condition and treatment. Now is not the time for casualness. Answer each person's questions in a respectful way, even when the questions are inane or repetitive. A wonderful idea, even if not always practical, is to write down and give at least the spokesperson for the group your name and a number by which they can reach you (i.e., switchboard, pager number). Even if they do not use it, they will have a sense of security and the definite knowledge that you are a doctor who they want to care for their sick family member. It may even be advisable or necessary to involve the clergy and/or the ethics committee of the hospital.

Be sure to write the details of each encounter in the patient's chart.

11.3   The Difficult Colleague

The difficult colleague is most often a fellow house staff person in any specialty. The problems you may have often fall into one of the following categories: work ethic, knowledge, attitude, ethics, morality, and ego.

Unfortunately, you will often come in contact with individuals who violate one of the aforementioned categories, and this will offend you greatly. You did not ask to be placed with these individuals, but they profoundly affect you, your job, and often the quality of patient care. So, it is within your right and obligation to aid the situation in any way that you are able. Very often, a quiet conversation with the colleague will make him aware that others notice his aberrant behavior, and he will attempt to improve. Sometimes a small group of associates who note the same problem can have the same discussion. If all attempts at mediating this colleague's poor behavior fail and as a last resort, a more senior doctor must be informed. The situation should not be permitted to smolder, as you will become more and more frustrated, and you will withdraw completely from the individual, which also does not make for a comfortable work and study environment. Certainly, it is your obligation to follow this matter until it is resolved. Our profession does not well tolerate a deviant physician.

While we are on this subject, you might critically evaluate your own demeanor in an effort to determine whether you might be a difficult colleague.

11.4   Medical Students

Medical students are not immune to abuse from residents. Residents are not immune to aberrant behavior by medical students. In questioning hundreds of residents about the students that rotate with them, they say that in general students are lazy. Some of them are on a mandatory rotation that they do not want to be on. Some of them just don't know what to do on the rotation and become immobilized with frustration. On the other hand, some medical students claim that certain residents are just nasty, don't want to be bothered with them, and don't want to teach. Each group should evaluate themselves, and their position. Each should make a vigorous attempt to adapt. Each should reevaluate their primary mission.

11.5   The Difficult Attending

The difficult attending can be a problem for every house staff member. Frankly, there is often at least one in each department. Sometimes this person's less-than-exemplary behavior is directed towards one or two residents, and sometimes to the whole group. At times, it is directed to his own faculty members and partners. A lot could be written on this subject; however, in the final summation, there are only two things to be said. Either you do whatever is necessary to get on his good side, or you respectfully ignore his anger but not him. Of course, the former is better than the latter; however, it takes a lot of energy and thought to stay ethical, moral, respectful, and energized by your work in this sort of situation. The latter tactic takes a certain finesse, but when it works, it can often change the entire situation, and the attending may very well see the error of his ways. Always remember that in due time you will be out of that situation, and he will remain.

11.6   The Difficult Consultant

The difficult consultant bears mentioning only to warn you and to suggest a way of handling him. The difficult consultant may:

– Not be available when you need him.
– Not come when needed.
– Not come in a timely fashion.

– Not hit it off with your patient.
– Not adequately provide the consultation that you desire.
– Not write a report of the consultation immediately and legibly.
– Not call you with a report.
– Speak to you in a condescending tone.
– Have a less experienced doctor do the consultation when a more experienced consultant is necessary.
– Not perform to standards that you have set for yourself and that you desire for your patient.

If you are not satisfied with the quality of the consultation, then immediately call a more superior consultant. The next time that you require a consultation, try to have someone else do it.

There is always the option of trying to correct the improper nuances in the consultant by gently telling him how you would prefer things done. This will very often work to your benefit, and both of you will have learned a lesson.

As always, critically evaluate yourself and make sure that you are the kind of consultant that you would like to have for your loved ones.

11.7   The Difficult Hospital Personnel

Hospital personnel include everyone you have contact with in the hospital, with the exception of the doctors. Very simply, just be nice to them, and they will be nice to you. Show great respect and appreciation for whatever job they do. Remember that most often they are not well paid, have troubles of their own, and you are just transient; here today, gone tomorrow.

Thank them in any small way that you can. They must have respect for your position, and you must have even more respect for theirs.

If there is a serious problem with any of them, then gently call it to the attention of their superiors, and try to offer a remedial solution. Never verbally attack ancillary personnel.

Chapter 12
Documentation

"Anybody can make history. Only a great person can write it."

— Oscar Wilde

12.1 General

The careful and accurate completion of medical records is not only an important physician responsibility, but it is also mandatory. Developing good habits of record keeping in medicine serves seven essential purposes:

1. Your record is an *aide-memoire* when you next see the patient. In other words, it reminds you, with your much cluttered mind, who the patient is, what is wrong, and what is being done about it.
2. A clear, accurate note is a *guide for your colleagues* who may need a quick review when seeing the patient in the years to come, for continuity of care.
3. The *clinic summary* should be a concise summation of the many hours of thought, investigation, and consultation that were spent in attempting to unravel the patient's problem.
4. It is a record of all diagnostic terms that are required for *case retrieval* in clinical investigations. References to the original pathology reports are essential in all tumor cases.

L.D. Florman, *The Portable Medical Mentor: Training Success*, DOI 10.1007/978-3-319-09852-4_12,
© Springer International Publishing Switzerland 2015

5. It affords a ***justification of payment*** by third parties, particularly when significant diagnostic and treatment efforts have been made.
6. All medical record notations must be ***timed in compliance*** with medical staff by-laws. These by-laws are generally mandated by the rules of the JCAH (Joint Commission on Accreditation of Hospitals). Also, always clearly document when an attending physician transfers patient care to another physician.
7. The medical record is a ***legal document*** and may be used in courts of law. The medical record is the first item that an attorney looks to for any inadequacies, discrepancies, untruths, amateurisms, or lies.

Thus, incomplete or inaccurate records may endanger the patient, inconvenience future clinicians, delay or abrogate payment, relegate the record to oblivion for purposes of research, and serve the courts for any cause.

An accurate record of everything that you do concerning patient care is mandatory for the remainder of your career. This is often required not only by law or statute or local tradition, but also primarily and ultimately to provide better patient care. The basic thread throughout this chapter is to document honestly and completely.

Your attending staff and the faculty are ultimately responsible for every act of patient care and documentation that you perform.

It is very important to remember that all documentation, whether handwritten or computer generated, constitutes a legal article, and can be used in many forums (court, committees, institutions, government agencies) for or against you, your faculty, and your institution, and for and against the patient. Remember, if you did not document an event, then either it did not happen or one could say that it did not occur as you recalled it.

Your signature must be clearly legible. If it is not, then you must print your name beside the signature. You should always write your pager or cell phone number under your signature.

The use of abbreviations has become prevalent not only in documentation, but also in presentations and casual medical talk. Acronyms can often become confusing, misleading, and dangerous, and they are not always universally recognizable. Most institutions have a list of acceptable abbreviations, and the Joint Commission for Accreditation of Hospitals constantly updates a comprehensive list on their website.

12.2   Patient Charts

12.2.1   History and Physical Examination

The correct format for performing and recording the results of the history and physical examination is learned in medical school and should be strictly adhered to. The history must be thorough, including not only significant items, but also those seemingly insignificant medical events that may be totally unrelated to the present illness. When documenting the diagnosis or impression, try not to use superlatives or adjectives, for example, "huge ventral hernia," "large wound of the buttocks," and "foul smelling sore of the left big toe." Instead, the correct terminology for the diagnosis should be written as "ventral hernia—10 cm × 20 cm," "wound of buttocks—24 cm × 12 cm," and "infected wound left big toe." The superlatives and adjectives may be used in the description part of the physical examination. Do not use street terms at all, like "bad scrape to leg" and "really high blood pressure."

Be sure to complete all of the blanks. It is impossible to know what organ system may become a problem during the hospitalization, and without a baseline examination, it will be difficult to provide adequate care.

If you are in charge of a particular patient, and a student or a person with less experience has written the history and physical examination, you should first check it in detail and then countersign it. A students' work must always be countersigned immediately.

12.2.2   Progress Notes

Progress notes should be written at least once a day, and more frequently if necessary. A note should be written during each and every visit. Include the date and time of each visit. A helpful, appreciated suggestion is to also print your specialty beside the date and time. Record all salient facts of the visit, as well as any change in the patient's condition, whether good or bad. Write any new or changed laboratory or test values, as well as the results of pathology or X-ray reports. Be very specific and very thorough. Sign your name legibly, and also print it if necessary. Never use a stamp. Always write or record the progress note directly after seeing the patient. Never write a progress note until you have personally seen and examined the patient.

It is a good idea to occasionally tabulate certain events when they are salient, for example, record of a temperature chart of the past few days in a patient with a fever or hemoglobin levels for the past few days in a patient who may be bleeding. There is nothing wrong with being innovative in the progress notes to help others who are reading the notes and in order to document that you know all of the events that have occurred.

12.2.3   Consultations

1. You Request the Consultation
   Consultations are usually requested of and by more senior residents and fellows, which implies a greater experience in diagnosis and treatment, and in note writing, which may or may not be true. Consultation requests should be made on a personal basis (i.e., telephone call), as well as a written order. The rules for the request are the following:
   - Write legibly.
   - State the precise reason for the consultation.
   - State the history as it pertains to the consultation.
   - State the results of your physical examination as it pertains to the consultation request.
   - State any salient laboratory or diagnostic results.

- If warranted, your request may also provide permission for the consultant to request any tests or perform whatever treatment found to be necessary.
- The request should be communicated directly to the consultant.

2. You Are the Consultant

- Respond as soon as possible.
- Do not send a more junior consultant than yourself.
- Familiarize yourself with the patient's chart.
- Examine the patient without undermining or contesting any diagnosis or treatments that the referring doctor has given.
- If appropriate, tell the patient what you are thinking, but that his doctor will explain it in detail.

Then, legibly write your diagnosis or impression <u>and</u> a detailed explanation. Suggest any changes in the treatment plan, but do not actually write orders for the changes, unless specifically instructed to do so by the referring doctor.

Regardless of what you think, or how you would handle the case, you must immediately speak to the referring doctor regarding your thoughts about the patient's condition and treatment. This task should not be left to a more junior person. Restrain from refuting the referring doctor in writing until you have had a chance to speak with him directly, as very often a "meeting of the minds" will come to an agreed-upon plan for the patient's overall benefit.

If additional specialty consultations are necessary, it is the referring doctor who must request them. If appropriate, and if desired by the referring doctor, you should follow the patient with at least daily visits until your services are no longer needed, and you have signed off on the case.

12.2.4   Orders

Writing accurate and legible orders can make the difference between life and death. All orders must be signed with the date and time and your pager number. Be very careful to use only approved abbreviations. For clarity, you should print the name of medications and their dose. Always print the route for the drug to be administered. Any complicated orders should be reviewed in person with the nurse who is in charge of the patient. Any "stat" orders should be directly identified to the nurse, not the ward secretary. Do not leave anything to chance when writing orders. Check and double-check them. <u>Students may not sign orders</u>.

12.2.5   Operation Reports

12.2.5.1   Preoperative Note

The operating surgeon is responsible for a handwritten pre-operative note on the day of the operation. This should include the following:

Preoperative Note

1. Diagnosis and short history.
2. Cardiorespiratory status with test results.
3. Laboratory data.
4. Consultations (if applicable).
5. Special studies (if applicable).
6. Indications for operation.
7. Surgical procedure proposed.
8. Operation permit consent: A statement should be included to the effect that the indications for operation, the type of surgical procedure, its implications, and possible complications have been discussed with the patient and understood, and that the patient agrees. Also note that their questions were answered.
9. Medications.
10. Blood available (if applicable).
11. Surgeons: The names of the attending surgeons should be provided with a statement that the case was discussed, and there was agreement on the plan of action.
12. Family: If appropriate, and if the patient desires, family members should be briefed at this point. This discussion

should be noted. Note who was present, preferably name and relationship.
13. Living will/advanced directives: The chart should be inspected for completeness of these two items.

12.2.5.2   Operative Report

The decision as to who will dictate the operative report should be made by the end of the operation. If you do the major part of the procedure, then you should dictate it; however, some attendings prefer to complete this task themselves. When possible listen to the attending dictating the report.

It must be noted whether the attending surgeon was present for the "key and critical portions of the procedure." This note is important not only for legal reasons but also for reimbursement purposes as well.

The dictated operative report has many purposes, all very important. It must be very complete and very accurate. This document will be referred to by other doctors, nurses, billing personnel, insurance companies, regulatory agencies, hospitals, compliance committees, peer-review organizations, lawyers, and your specialty examining board. It is a valuable teaching and research tool. The following is a good format for dictating:

Operative Note

1. Name of person dictating.
2. Name of patient: Essential patient information to properly track the patient.
3. Patient identification number.
4. Date of surgery.
5. Date dictated.
6. Name of surgeon(s).
7. Name of assistant(s).
8. Preoperative diagnosis: Not to be overstated, reason for performing the surgical procedures.
9. Postoperative diagnosis: The pre- and post-diagnosis should conform to ICD-10 coding.

10. Title of operation(s): A comprehensive and accurate list and description of services provided during the operative setting; each procedure should approximate a known CPT code; note the size of a lesion, the size of the excision, and the depth of the excision; note size and precise location of all lacerations individually.
11. Indications for surgery: This will aid the billing department and the reviewers.
12. Type of anesthesia.
13. Description of operation: In-depth description of the entire operative setting, which must support the diagnoses, the procedural listings, and the indications; it should be noted whether the procedure was more difficult, bilateral, and lengthy; indicate all layers of closure; if the wound was not closed, this should be explicitly mentioned; clearly indicate partial or complete excision (hemicolectomy vs. total colectomy); the correct side of the body should be indicated and consistent throughout. No abbreviation. No street language. Only real medical terms. Only real anatomy language.
14. Findings at operation.
15. Complications.
16. Drains and catheters.
17. Estimated blood loss.
18. Total fluid replacement and type.

Do not use superlatives; just be factual. Make it so clear and informative that a doctor reading it 20 years from now will have no questions, nor will a peer reviewer have a problem interpreting it. It is mandatory that you dictate the operative report directly following the procedure.

Here are some things that should not be in an operative note:

"The arms were carefully tucked to the patient's sides"
"The elevator was carefully placed in the mouth"
"The vein was dissected with great difficulty"
"Extra time was necessary to get a new blade"
"I took time to elevate the periosteum"
"Pre-op Diagnosis: Road rash of arms"

12.2.5.3   Postoperative Note

An "op note" should be written in the progress notes at the end of the operation, so that recovery room staff and floor nurses will know what has been done to their patient prior to receiving the dictated report. This should be simple and complete:

Postoperative Note

1. Date, service
2. Heading: "OP NOTE"
3. Name of surgeon
4. Name of assistant
5. Preoperative diagnosis
6. Postoperative diagnosis
7. Operation
8. Anesthesia
9. Findings
10. Complications
11. Drains
12. Estimated blood loss
13. Signature and pager number

12.2.6   Discharge Summary

The discharge summary is usually dictated, but can be hand-written. This important record must not be delegated to medical students or members of the medical team who are not familiar with the case. The format is as follows:

Discharge Summary

1. Date of admission
2. Date of discharge
3. Chief complaint
4. History of present illness
5. Hospital course
6. Procedures performed with dates
7. Laboratory tests done and results (only when directly related to diagnosis)

8. Special tests (only when related to diagnosis)
9. X-ray and pathology descriptions
10. Medications
11. Blood received
12. Daily trends in temperature, blood pressure, etc.
13. Complications of hospitalization
14. Discharge condition
15. Discharge disposition
16. Discharge medications, diet, activities
17. Follow-up (very specific, i.e., who, when, where)
18. Final diagnosis (list all of them)
19. Signature

12.2.7   Informed Consent

Informed consent is the legal and ethical right that a patient has to be fully informed about his condition and treatments so that the patient can participate in all of the phases and choices concerning his or her health care. The physician has an ethical and a legal duty to inform the patient in language the patient can understand, so the patient can decide what is best.

A complete informed consent must include the following elements:

• The nature of the treatment or procedure.
• Reasonable alternatives to the proposed treatment.
• The relevant risks, benefits, and uncertainties relating to each alternative.
• Assessment of the patient understanding.
• The acceptance of the treatment by the patient.

Many books have been written on informed consent, and controversy will shroud the concept for a long time to come. However, the intern and resident must become an expert on this subject by the first time he or she finds himself or herself before the patient or the family in a situation of explaining and requesting informed consent.

It will be obvious to you that no two situations will be the same, and neither will any two informed consents be the same. However, in every situation, you must adhere to the basic concepts, which are:

- Nature and seriousness of the treatment or procedure.
- Alternatives to the treatment or procedure.
- Risks, benefits, and uncertainties of the treatment or procedure.

When special circumstances arise, there are special remedies for all of them, and the correct protocol must be observed. When in doubt, call upon the nursing supervisor or your attending for help.

12.2.8   DNR

Do not resuscitate orders that appear to throw a cloud over a patient's chart. Similar to other medical decisions, the decision to attempt to retrieve the life of a patient who suffers from cardiopulmonary arrest involves a very careful consideration of the potential likelihood for clinical benefit, taking into account the patient's general physical condition, his prognosis, and his preferences for the intervention and its likely outcome.

I will not delve into all of the nuances and examples of DNR and CPR. Most institutions have policies about this subject, and usually well-written protocols. You should become very familiar with them very early in your training.

12.2.9   Living Will

In 1991, the federal government enacted the *Patient Self-Determination Act*, requiring that patients be informed about their right to participate in healthcare decisions, including their right to have an advance directive. Advance directives are broken down into two broad categories: instructive and proxy. The *Living Will* is one type of instructive directive; however, there are others such as no transfusion and no CPR.

The proxy directive is generally a *Durable Power of Attorney for Health Care*, which permits the designation of a surrogate medical decision maker of the patient's choosing. This surrogate is empowered to make all medical decisions for the patient, in the event he or she is incapacitated.

All hospitals ask each patient whether they have a living will. If they do not, they are given the opportunity to have one on the spot.

You should be familiar with your patient's living will. If a surrogate has been appointed, and your patient is incapacitated, then you must treat the surrogate as though he was the patient, for matters of informed consent.

12.2.10   Prescriptions

Use the standard hospital prescription form. Fill it out completely and legibly. It is good practice to print the entire prescription so that no errors in interpretation are possible. Following your signature, print your name and pager number (with area code). Make sure that you circle the maximum number of pills to prescribe, as well as the refill/no refill space.

Always record the prescription as well as any refills in the patient's chart. Be very careful to whom you give the prescription. Be vigilant with those patients requesting refills for narcotics or mood-changing medications. Do not leave prescription pads lying around.

12.2.11   Letters, Authorizations, Status Reports

You will frequently be called upon to write letters for patients. If the request is legitimate, you should graciously do it. If you determine that it is nonsense, then just tell the patient that you are unable to comply with his request.

Authorizations for durable medical equipment often require a letter from you. This should be done quickly, as the patient is most likely in immediate need.

Insurance companies, home health agencies, and governmental agencies, for instance, frequently request status reports and forms on patients. This is usually presented to you by means of a standard form for you to fill in the blanks. These forms should be completed with the patient's chart in front of you. Be honest and complete.

A last word about your written notes: If you need to correct something in any written medical document at a later point, under no circumstance should you erase it, black it out, scratch it out, or white it out. Place one line through it, so that it can still be read, place the date and your initials adjacent to it, and write a new note, or an addendum at the bottom. Do not write the new note in the margins or between lines.

Chapter 13
Presentations

"You don't have to be a chicken to make an omelet."

—Mark Twain

"Don't let it end like this. Tell them I said something."

—last words of Pancho Villa

You will often be called upon to make presentations, sometimes to small groups and not infrequently to large and austere groups. It behooves you to use the small group presentations to perfect and streamline your technique in preparation and delivery so that your large and/or important group presentations will be very professional. Formal presentations are an art form. A really good one is as enjoyable to present as it is to receive. Once you make the presentation, store it away for the next time. The following are suggestions to facilitate your preparation and presentation.

13.1 Preparation of Slides

1. Use PowerPoint.
2. Don't be too concerned with slide backgrounds, intricate title slides, animations, or fancy graphics; they can distract from your presentation.

L.D. Florman, *The Portable Medical Mentor: Training Success*, DOI 10.1007/978-3-319-09852-4_13,
© Springer International Publishing Switzerland 2015

3. Use only one font. No fancy fonts.
4. No light print like yellow or pink.
5. Use footnotes. Give credit where credit is due.
6. Try to integrate into your presentation, and give credit to any work done by your attendings, the department, and/or the institution. Graphs must be uncomplicated but detailed enough for the audience to quickly interpret them.
7. Charts should not have a lot of barely readable numbers, but should be reduced to their essence, and placed in big print.
8. No complicated tables or charts.
9. Adjust the complexity and the language of the presentation to the audience, i.e., students, residents, attendings, nurses, lay public, etc.
10. You and a friend should review the entire presentation, double-checking the spelling and order of the slides.
11. Keep in mind that slides are only an adjunct to your presentation. You are the focus of attention. Use the slides to enlighten the audience, and more important to make your verbal presentation flow.

13.2   Presentation

1. Arrive early.
2. Order needed equipment in advance, and make sure it works. Make sure you know how to operate it.
3. Try using some sort of "memory stick" rather than a CD. It's a lot cooler! It is always a good idea to have a backup disk with you.
4. Dress for the occasion. It shows, and commands respect.
5. Stand up; regardless of how many presentations you have seen where the presenter is seated.
6. Don't lean against anything.
7. Keep your hands out of your pockets.
8. Use a laser pointer if available.
9. Look at your audience. Don't ever look at the floor, or the ceiling.

10. Don't rub your chin or cover your mouth with your hand. This gives the body language of lying.
11. Only look at the screen for brief intervals.
12. Do not read from the slides. Your audience will be reading them. It is disconcerting to repeat what they are reading.
13. Don't cross your arm in front of your body when pointing to the screen. Use the hand closest to the screen.
14. Never apologize for a bad slide. If the slide is bad, don't use it.
15. A certain amount of humor is permitted as long as it is in context.
16. Ask for questions or comments. Be prepared to answer.
17. At the end, simply say "thank you."

Chapter 14
Mortality and Morbidity Conference

"If you get all the facts, your judgment can be right; if you don't get all the facts, it can't be right."

—Bernard M. Baruch

"Tell me and I forget. Show me and I remember Teach me and I learn."

—Benjamin Franklin

14.1 Background

The Mortality and Morbidity Conference (M&M) is certainly the most important hour of the week for students, residents, and their teachers. Here is the last bastion of medical intellect, competition, showmanship, and debate. And, the most important component in the M&M is the absolutely perfect presentation, which requires extensive preparation, and the honest willingness to accept blame, and/or severe criticism.

14.2 Preparation

(a) Collect all of the facts of the case. If certain historical information is not readily available, search it out. If necessary, call previous doctors, clinics, hospitals, and, if

L.D. Florman, *The Portable Medical Mentor: Training Success*, DOI 10.1007/978-3-319-09852-4_14, © Springer International Publishing Switzerland 2015

appropriate, the patient's family. The data, regardless of how trivial, must be sought.

(b) Discuss the case to be presented with your attending. This is not only a matter of courtesy, but it may also give you additional, detailed information, and it will also prevent you from getting blindsided by questions from that attending. If the attending for that case cannot be present for the conference, the case should not be presented.

(c) Only residents who thoroughly know the case, the main issues, and the controversies surrounding the complication should be presenting. Thus, the case should be presented by the most senior resident who will conduct himself as if he were the attending surgeon and the patient was from his private office.

14.3   Presentation

Each institution's M&M conference has its little idiosyncrasies not limited to specific seating arrangements, attendance, and the precise way in which the case is presented. While some (very few) places do not take the conference very seriously, you have the opportunity to elevate it to a new level by preparing your presentation in the following format.

(a) Prepare a brief, **printed summary** to serve as a sort of "database." Do not waste time reviewing facts. The audience will have more time to formulate its thoughts and questions. Include line drawings if applicable.

(b) Have **audiovisual aids** available (overhead projector, PowerPoint, microscope projector, etc.). A picture is worth a 1,000 words, and it certainly makes your discussion more objective.

(c) **Dress** for the occasion. Carry yourself as though you were the professor. Review the chapter on "Presentations."

(d) Even though the surgical operation is probably the central event, it is not necessarily the most important event. Present a very clear, specific, and anatomically precise description of the **technical operation and the findings at the time of surgery**.

(e) Attempt to anticipate the **questions** you might be asked, and incorporate the answers into your presentation.

(f) **Avoid the use of terms** like "extremely difficult," "massive," "odd looking," "weird," and "never seen that before." This is not the time for subjectivity. What is exaggerated for some may be commonplace for others.

(g) Review **X-rays** with the radiologist, and better yet, have the radiologist attend the conference. Never tell the audience that you could not get the X-rays.

(h) Do not waste the audience's time telling them of **laboratory values**. Write them on the blackboard, or better, include them in a printed handout at the beginning of the presentation.

(i) The M&M should be fun (we surgeons are a morbid bunch). The dynamic of the meeting is the interplay between the knowledge and the ignorance of both the residents and the audience. Inappropriate questions as well as inappropriate answers determine who walks out with their heads held high. Therefore, **rehearse your presentation** with your fellow residents and/or your attending.

(j) Following your immaculate presentation, there will be a dedicated time for **questions**.

1. Be polite. Show respect to the questioner, even if the question is dumb and shows a complete lack of understanding of the case.

2. You may say "I don't know." If you believe that somebody else in the room knows the answer, you may ask them to respond, but do not put them on the spot if the answer is going to be another "I don't know."

3. If you are well prepared and your presentation is complete, the questions will be directed at your thought process rather than the details of the case.

(k) Put the **case in context** with the known and generally accepted practice of the art of medicine. Cite references from recognized and not-so-recognized authorities on the subject, both for and against the evaluation and treatment of the patient in question. The literature you cite may be an ally or an enemy. It should be presented in a balanced format.

4. The **summary of the case** and its complications should be short, honest, and sometimes humbling. This is where an admission of guilt is made if necessary. It is in this closing statement where those in the room will or will not see the fruits of their labors in helping to create a mature physician.

(l) Finally, the **attending** should respectfully be called upon for comment. Most likely, she has been quite vocal throughout, but she should have a dedicated moment to have the last word.

The purpose of the M&M conference is to teach and learn. The proceedings are protected from disclosure in court, and therefore unabashed honesty is demanded and expected. There should be no attempt to cover up for or to protect anybody.

This has been only a brief description and a few suggestions to make your presentation at the M&M conference more effective. There are entire books on the subject. We suggest reading "Gordon's Guide to the Surgical Morbidity and Mortality Conference," by Leo A. Gordon, M.D. (Hanley & Belfus, Inc., Mosby).

Chapter 15
On Call

"Sleep is a symptom of caffeine deprivation"

— Author unknown

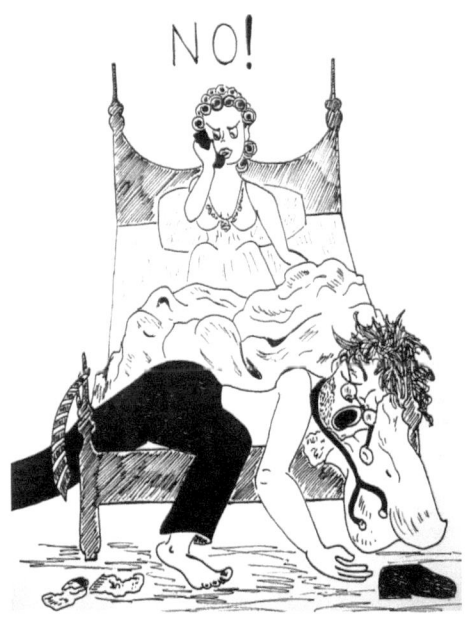

Fig. 15.1.   On call at home

L.D. Florman, *The Portable Medical Mentor:*
Training Success, DOI 10.1007/978-3-319-09852-4_15,
© Springer International Publishing Switzerland 2015

Complaining about being on call serves no useful purpose. Just take it on the chin and go about your business. Learn to love it. This is what you signed up for, so don't dread it… embrace it!

15.1   On Call in the Hospital

On call in the hospital can be one of those necessary evils, if you permit it to be. Being that it is necessary evil, why not make the most of it? This time spent away from family, friends, and your own bed gives you several opportunities:

(a) A time to study.
(b) An opportunity to learn in real emergency situations, without the convenience and relative safety of attending staff and numerous residents.
(c) An opportunity to do more difficult surgical cases, and see more complex medical situations.
(d) An opportunity to learn when tired.

15.2   At Home Call

Taking call from home can be stifling. It is better to treat this as though you were in the hospital. Relax, study, and be ever ready to go to the hospital at a moment's notice. No Alcohol. No rowdy parties where you won't hear the cell phone. Better to not get into any dirty home projects. Be within easy driving range. Don't have any important company over who might be disappointed when you have to leave.

Timely, accurate, and complete hand-offs are now mandatory (ACGME). They serve a very useful purpose. Do not take them nonchalantly.

Chapter 16
Family and Friends

Happiness is having a large, loving, close-knit family in another city.

—George Burns (1896–1996)

Most nonmedical people haven't the vaguest idea exactly what you do at the hospital. You bring home a lot of juicy stories, you are tired and irritable, but family and friends are unaware of the intricacies of your job and the huge commitment you have undertaken. You are seeing many things that few are privy to. Perhaps you are more peaceful with yourself. Life seems to hold a different meaning. It is impossible to be around sickness and disease all day, and not be changed in many ways. People notice the conversion that you are going through, but they don't quite understand it. It certainly would not be a bad idea to permit those closest to you (spouse, significant other, mother, etc.) to read this book as an aid to appreciating what you are going through, to understanding your commitment both in time and energy, and to help them comprehend your possible mood swings.

Your immediate family is going to suffer during your training. They have already probably come to understand your time obligation. Even at home, you will have little time for family niceties. So, be very cognizant that you are not the only one in distress. Be very jealous of your time with your family

L.D. Florman, *The Portable Medical Mentor: Training Success*, DOI 10.1007/978-3-319-09852-4_16, © Springer International Publishing Switzerland 2015

and friends. Build that time into your daily and weekly routine, and make it high quality.

A word about "medical secrets" is in order. It's acceptable to tell family and friends about interesting things that happen in the hospital, but be very careful not to be too specific. Breaches in HIPAA (see Chap. 24) can get you fired, and a lot worse come with significant financial penalties. Telling stories about your attendings by name or reference, your colleagues, the institution, or the patients can come back at you in ways that you cannot dream of. Although you may seem to be a more interesting person when you tell these stories, remain professional and generic in recounting them.

Chapter 17
Your Health

"Happiness is nothing more than good health and a bad memory."

— Albert Schweitzer

Medical school and residency place unusual demands on your life, both mentally and physically. It is a burden on your entire system and can be truly overwhelming. Residency as well as the clinical years of medical school thrust you into the real world of disease, trauma, life, and death, and <u>you</u> are making the medical decisions. Having this responsibility can be both exhilarating and depressing. These extremes of feelings will eventually lessen with time and experience, but that is not to say that they will or should become blunted. As you learn to internalize and, at will, externalize these feelings, you will develop a healthier mind and more mature compassion.

In an effort to give your mind every opportunity to function correctly, it is mandatory that your body is healthy. You could consciously strengthen your mind or your psyche; however, your body is always at your beck and call, just waiting to be strengthened, or weakened. When your body is kept in good condition, your mind has less to contend with.

As difficult as it may seem, you should place yourself on a regular **physical fitness program**. Of course, you have time! Right? Make and take the time, as it is very important for you, your family, and your patients to have not only an intelligent doctor, but one who exemplifies good health. Here are some ideas to get you started:

If you are already on a program of exercise, continue it.

Join a fitness center. The hospital often has special prices at a center, and, if associated with a university, it could be free of charge.

Use the stairs for one to three flights.

If practical, walk to and from your home.

Ride a bike to work, on the weekends, or anytime.

Take long walks. Gradually lengthen your distance to 3–4 miles a day, three to four times per week.

Get up a regular basketball, football, or volleyball game.

Ask somebody to buy you a treadmill.

The important thing is to be consistent in your effort, even when you do not feel like expending much energy.

Residency brings with it a whole new **eating** agenda, and the associated problems of eating too much, not enough, or not correctly. Here are some suggestions:

If you are grossly overweight, lose weight. Easy for us to say. But now there are so many good weight loss programs that work, you should be able to trim yourself down rather easily. Obesity does not engender patient confidence.

No donuts in the doctors' lounge.

Try a bagel (no cream cheese) in the morning.

No fast food. Not even in a pinch. If you must indulge, most fast food places have some dietetic items on the menu.

Cut down on fat and calories, but do it consistently.

No fad diets. You can't afford to take a chance on the metabolic changes they can induce. Consult the hospital dietician.

No in-between meals munching.

One more health issue is also important. Much of your mental and physical health is determined by how much **fun** you have. Permit yourself the gift of having fun when it is appropriate. This includes time-outs, when you relinquish the trials and tribulations of being in charge of human life.

It is cleansing, purifying, and just plain relaxing to regularly be with family and friends, go to a movie, or just take it easy with a good book. It is likewise important to be able to laugh, and enjoy it, and be humorous, and be enjoyed by others.

Dr. Florman's creed:

- Laugh when it's funny.
- Cry when it's sad.
- Joke when appropriate.
- Be serious when serious is necessary
- Be happy all of the time. You should be happy; just look at where you are and what you have accomplished.

Chapter 18
Medical-Legal

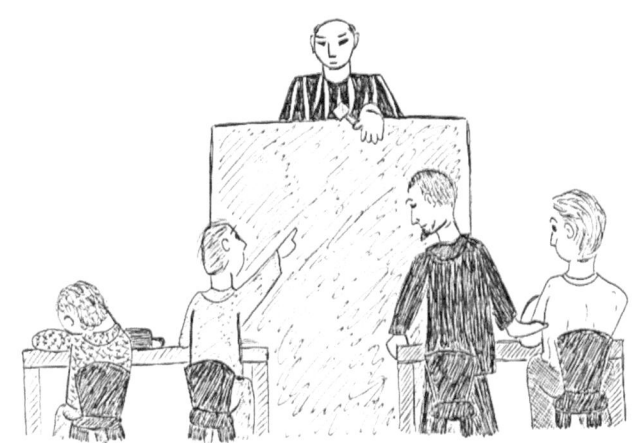

<small>Fig. 18.1. The Courtroom</small>

> *"Becoming involved in a law suit is like being*
> *ground to bits in a slow mill; it's being roasted at a*
> *slow fire; it's being stung to death by a single bee; it's*
> *being drowned by drops; it's going mad by grains.*
> *Hundreds of thousands of people are exposed to*
> *such torture each year, some of them actually*
> *choosing to initiate the process. They invariably find*
> *the experience painful, protracted and expensive.*

L.D. Florman, *The Portable Medical Mentor:* 103
Training Success, DOI 10.1007/978-3-319-09852-4_18,
© Springer International Publishing Switzerland 2015

> *When it has run its course, they often realize that it*
> *was futile. Yet there remains a queue of victims*
> *impatient for their turn."*

—Charles Dickens

18.1   Malpractice

Unfortunately, most likely you will one day be sued. It might be something that you did wrong. It might be due to something somebody else did wrong. It could be due to a lack of communication between you and the patient. It could be due to a patient or their family just looking for a bunch of money. The reasons are endless. Remember, these lawsuits cost the patients nothing. The plaintiff's lawyers work on a contingency. The defendants' lawyers get paid from the beginning.

Malpractice is defined as "treatment which is contrary to accepted medical standards and which produces injurious results in patients." Since most medical malpractice actions are based on laws governing negligence, the law recognizes that medicine is an inexact art and that there can be no absolute liability. Thus, the cause of action is usually "failure" of the defendant and/or physician to exercise that reasonable degree of skill, learning, care, and treatment ordinarily possessed by others of the same profession in the community.

Not only is the definition confusing and open-ended to the average physician, the entire process can become unnerving for not only the physician, but also for the purported victim as well. For many reasons, it will make your life much easier if you can avoid the malpractice system. To keep yourself out of trouble, you must practice medicine as though trouble were right around the corner, virtually for the rest of your life.

Briefly, here are some rough guidelines to live by in order to stay out of the courtroom:

- Do not practice medicine beyond the scope of your abilities and level of training.
- Write notes clearly, legibly, and contemporaneously. Include your signature, the date, and time.

- Be thorough, noting positive and negative findings.
- Record in the chart every patient visit and family member discussion.
- Double check your written orders.
- Fill in all of the blanks on forms.
- Use only recognized abbreviations.
- Obtain adequate informed consent, preferably witnessed by others.
- Never, ever, alter medical records. Corrections can be made as a separate entry, signed and dated. Never write between the lines or in the margins.
- All written and called-in prescriptions must be entered into the patient's chart.
- All telephone calls from or about a patient should be noted in the patient's chart.
- Respond quickly to patients' concerns and telephone calls.
- Always be available.
- Remember HIPAA.
- If you err in any way, discuss it with the patient.
- Be honest. Be compassionate.

18.2   Legal Documents

Just about everything that you write or type into a computer during your training could be considered a legal document, and therefore could be admissible in court. The patient's medical record is certainly a legal document and requires great care and forethought when written. Once entered into the chart, it cannot be removed or altered, except by very explicit means. And even those means still leave the original writings intact and visible.

Keep in mind that whenever a patient goes to a lawyer with a complaint about you, the first thing that lawyer will do will be to get a copy of the complete medical record. He/she will scrupulously dissect it and pick out weaknesses that will astound you. From those weaknesses in the record he/she will make you look like a total uncaring, untrustworthy, uneducated, inept, uncompassionate, moronic individual.

18.3   Responding to a Subpoena or Requests from Attorneys

If you should receive a subpoena to produce documents, or any other request for a medical record, you must immediately and personally give it to the legal affairs department of the hospital. Note in your little black book the date and time and who it was handed to. Under no circumstance should you neglect it, delay it, or respond yourself. The failure to timely comply with a subpoena could place you in contempt of court, with subsequent fine and/or imprisonment.

A request from an attorney for information about a patient must also be immediately given to the legal department for disposition. You are also required to give a copy of the letter to the chairman of your department. Do not give it to anyone else. Do not talk to anyone about it. This is very important. Keep your mouth shut. These letters often appear quite benign, but could be the beginning of a lot of grief for you.

18.4   Testifying

It is very possible that you will be called to testify as a witness in a deposition or trial about a patient who you somehow came in contact with. The legal department will help you with this. Unfortunately, this is a necessary, unwanted part of your education. The only thing you have to do is be honest, knowledgeable, believable, and compassionate.

There is not enough room in this book to give the subject of testifying any justice. However, you can prepare yourself for the inevitable time when you will be called upon to testify for either the prosecution, the defense, or for yourself. When that time arrives, your attorney will prepare you for the occasion. The purpose here is to encourage you to begin thinking towards that fateful time and to return to this section occasionally to reinforce the way you should behave in a court of law. These suggestions and observations could help you one day.

- Few things will cause you more anger, frustration, and anxiety than dealing with an attorney.
- Keep your "cool" when dealing with attorneys.
- Jurors do not like hotheads or smart alecks.
- Always be the nicest person in the room. Judges and jurors like pleasant witnesses.
- A good witness is a teacher.
- Study your testimony and chart as you would your most important final exam.
- Never promise a result to a patient. The promise may be repeated to you in court.
- Do not try to impress the attorneys or jury with your importance.
- Dress for court as you would for an important interview. Look clean, pressed, and professional. Shine your shoes. No fancy watches or jewelry.
- Make eye contact with the attorneys, judge, and jury.
- It is better to say "I don't know." No lying. No wavering.
- Do not fidget. Keep your hands off your face. Never look at the floor or ceiling.
- For video testimony, look at the camera when speaking.
- Use plain English. Stay away from medical terminology or abbreviations that the jury will not understand.
- Watch out for convoluted, compound, or trick questions.
- Do not carry a medical textbook into court or to a deposition. Anything in the book can be used.
- If an attorney quotes your prior depositions or some medical literature, you have the right to see the entire text. Beware of statements taken out of context.
- Answer to the lawyer; explain to the jury.
- Juries love pictures and diagrams. Use them liberally. Ask the judge if you can step down from the stand to explain or demonstrate a point. Juries like that also.
- When asked to respond to a hypothetical question, be absolutely sure it fits the facts of the case.
- Do not use language (terminology) unless you know the definition. You can count on the attorney asking you to define terms such as "sensitivity" or "specificity."

- If you attribute a disease or injury to a cause, be sure you are correct, and it is supported by the peer-reviewed literature.
- Know the facts of every case you are involved in. Someday you may have to explain the diagnosis and treatment to a group of nonmedical strangers (a jury).
- For the purpose of testimony, symptoms do not equal a diagnosis.
- Be sure you know the patient's chart in great detail before any testimony. Read your notes.
- Be sure you know the literature on the topic before you give testimony.
- Ask your attorney to explain the legal facts of the case to you. If you do not understand, ask him again.
- If you are presented with a summons stating that you are party to a lawsuit, keep your mouth shut. Discuss it only with your chairman and the legal department. There is one exception to this rule: You may discuss it with your personal attorney. If you find it necessary to retain a personal attorney, he or she should be a litigator who is very familiar with medical malpractice.
- Never fail to disclose on any employment application that you were named in a case, even if the case was dropped. Read the application questions carefully, and answer honestly. If you have survived a lawsuit, have an attorney help you draw up a letter of explanation of what happened. Keep this letter forever; you will have to use it to explain disclosure in future employment applications.

18.5   Conflict of Interest

During your training, there will be opportunities to accept gifts from vendors, patients, students, etc. The rules pertaining to this vary among institutions. The laws of some states and the Federal laws are quite specific and should be researched. As a rule of thumb, do not accept anything from anybody in exchange for favors or for the use of a product. That should keep you out of trouble.

18.6   Child Abuse

Child abuse takes many forms, including child sexual abuse, pedophilia, physical abuse, neglect, emotional neglect, failure to thrive, and Munchausen by Proxy Syndrome. Interns and residents, and physicians in general, are in a position daily to discern these travesties on children. Most states mandate that physicians must, by law, report to the authorities these aberrant acts. The possibility of child abuse must be constantly in the back of your mind. If you suspect you have seen the results of such an act, you should either consult a nursing supervisor before telephoning the police, or just call the police. The law will protect any person who reports child abuse, so long as the report is not made with malice of intent.

The laws are less specific for elder abuse; however, it should always be a question in your mind when treating debilitated older patients.

Chapter 19
The System

"I must create a system, or be enslaved by another man's."

— William Blake

The System refers to the rules, regulations, and laws that guide us, making us better physicians, protecting our patients, and weeding out the occasional, inappropriate physician. Throughout your career you will be subjected to various regulatory and certification organizations. You might find some of them cumbersome; however, they are necessary, and their effectiveness has for the most part withstood the test of time. Eight of these organizations which most profoundly and very personally affect you from medical school to the end of your formal training and beyond are:

- LCME: Liaison Committee on Medical Education
- ACGME: Accreditation Council for Graduate Medical Education
- AAMC: Association of American Medical Colleges
- USMLE: United States Medical Licensing Examination
- NBME: National Board of Medical Examiners
- NRMP: National Residency Matching Program
- ABMS: American Board of Medical Specialties
- ECFMG: Educational Council for Foreign Medical Graduates

L.D. Florman, *The Portable Medical Mentor: Training Success*, DOI 10.1007/978-3-319-09852-4_19,
© Springer International Publishing Switzerland 2015

You should become familiar with each of these. Some of them are more important in the early years, and could have very little to do with your final career life. Others will be with you for a very long time as they regulate the practice of medicine.

It is beyond the scope of this book to give the attention that each of the above deserves. The initials will keep reappearing in your life throughout your career

19.1   Liaison Committee on Medical Education

Medical education programs leading to the MD degree in the United States and Canada are accredited by the Liaison Committee on Medical Education (LCME). The LCME's scope is limited to complete and independent medical education programs whose students are geographically located in the United States or Canada for their education and that are operated by universities or medical schools chartered in the United States or Canada.

LCME accreditation is a voluntary, peer-review process of quality assurance that determines whether the program meets established standards. Programs are required to demonstrate that their graduates exhibit general professional competencies that are appropriate for entry to the next stage of their training and that serve as the foundation for lifelong learning and proficient medical care. While recognizing the existence and appropriateness of diverse institutional missions and educational objectives, the LCME subscribes to the proposition that local circumstances do not justify accreditation of a substandard program of medical education leading to the MD degree.

It is obvious that the LCME is of vital interest to medical students. It is recognized by the U.S. Department of Education as the reliable authority for the accreditation of medical schools leading to the MD degree. One of the more visible things that the LCME does is to mandate duty hour restrictions for medical students (Chap. 21).

19.2   Accreditation Committee on Graduate Medical Education

The Accreditation Council for Graduate Medical Education (ACGME) is an organization responsible for the accreditation of about 9,200 residency education programs in the United States. The ACGME's volume of accredited programs makes it one of the largest private accrediting agencies in the country, if not the world.

Stakeholders of the ACGME's accreditation process are residency programs, their sponsoring institutions, residents, medical students, the specialty boards of the American Board of Medical Specialties (ABMS), patients, payers, government, and the general public. Accreditation offers these stakeholders assurance that a given residency program and its sponsoring institutions meet an accepted set of educational standards. The ACGME accredits residency programs in 133 specialty and subspecialty areas of medicine, including all programs leading to primary Board certification by the 24 member boards of the American Board of Medical Specialties.

To develop and refine its accreditation standards and to review accredited programs for compliance with the standards, the ACGME relies on experts in the various medical specialties. Twenty-six specialty-specific committees, known as Residency Review Committees (RRCs), periodically initiate revision of the standards and review accredited programs in each specialty and its subspecialties.

The business of the ACGME is mostly applicable to residents and fellows. The duty hour rules are regulated by the ACGME (Chap. 21).

19.3   Association of American Medical Colleges

The AAMC has several wide reaching functions which will serve you for your entire career in training. The most important one for students is ERAS (Electronic Residency Application Service) which was developed to transmit residency applications via the Internet, including electronic transmittal of USMLE transcripts to residency programs which participate in ERAS. You will rapidly become an expert at this system when it is time to apply for residency position. Information on electronic transmittal of USMLE transcripts through ERAS is available for students and graduates of accredited medical schools in the United States and Canada from the medical schools. ERAS is available to students and graduates of medical schools outside the United States and Canada through the ECFMG.

19.4   National Board of Medical Examiners

The NBME develops and manages the USMLE. While the individual licensing boards grant the license to practice medicine, all medical boards in the United States accept a passing score on the USMLE as evidence that an applicant demonstrates the core competencies to practice medicine. As a result, healthcare consumers throughout the nation enjoy a high degree of confidence that their doctors have met a common standard. The NBME and the Federation of State Medical Boards co-sponsor the USMLE, and the Educational Commission for Foreign Medical Graduates is the third collaborator in the USMLE program.

19.5   United States Medical Licensing Examination

The USMLE is a three-step examination for medical licensure in the United States and is sponsored by the Federation of State Medical Boards (FSMB) and the National Board of Medical Examiners (NBME).

The USMLE assesses a physician's ability to apply knowledge, concepts, and principles, and to demonstrate fundamental patient-centered skills that are important in health and disease and that constitute the basis of safe and effective patient care.

Each of the three Steps of the USMLE complements the others; no Step can stand alone in the assessment of readiness for medical licensure.

19.5.1   Step 1

Assesses the examinee's understanding and ability to apply important concepts of the sciences basic to the practice of medicine, with special emphasis on principles and mechanisms underlying health, disease, and modes of therapy. Step 1 assesses your mastery of the sciences that provide a foundation for the safe and competent practice of medicine in the present, as well as the scientific principles required for the maintenance of competence through lifelong learning.

19.5.2   Step 2

Assesses the examinee's ability to apply medical knowledge, skills, and understanding of clinical science essential for the provision of patient care under supervision, with an emphasis on health promotion and disease prevention. Step 2 focuses on principles of clinical sciences and basic patient-centered skills that provide the foundation for the safe and competent practice of medicine.

The clinical skills examination is a separately administered component of Step 2 and is referred to as Step 2 Clinical Skills, or Step 2 CS. The computer-based, multiple-choice component of Step 2 is referred to as Step 2 Clinical Knowledge, or Step 2 CK.

USMLE Step 2 CS is administered at five regional test centers (CSEC Centers) in the United States.

19.5.3   Step 3

Assesses the examinee's understanding of biomedical and clinical science essential for the unsupervised practice of medicine, with an emphasis on patient management in ambulatory settings. Step 3 provides a final assessment of physicians assuming independent responsibility for delivering general medical care.

Your Step 1 score is all important. This is the first and quite often the most important parameter used by residency programs to evaluate your application. There are books written which tell you how to prepare for this test. There are thousands of sample questions available. Do not wait till the last minute, week, or month to prepare. The highest profile residencies and locations command the highest scores.

19.6   American Board of Medical Specialties

The American Board of Medical Specialties (ABMS) is an organization of medical specialty boards with shared goals and standards related to the certification of medical specialists. Certification includes initial specialty and subspecialty certification and maintenance of certification throughout the physician's career. The mission of the ABMS is to maintain and improve the quality of medical care by assisting the Member Boards in their efforts to develop and utilize professional and educational standards for the certification of physician specialists in the United States and internationally. The intent of both the initial certification of physicians and the maintenance of certification is to provide assurance to the public that a physician specialist certified by a Member Board of the ABMS has successfully completed an approved educational program and evaluation process which includes components designed to assess the medical knowledge, judgment, professionalism, and clinical and communication skills required to provide quality patient care in that specialty.

The ABMS serves to coordinate the activities of its Member Boards and to provide information to the public, the governments of the United States and other countries, the profession, and its Members concerning issues involving certification of physicians in the United States and internationally.

The official ABMS Member Boards and Associate Members are (year approved as an ABMS Member Board in parentheses):

- Allergy and Immunology
- Anesthesiology
- Colon and Rectal Surgery
- Dermatology
- Emergency Medicine
- Family Medicine
- Internal Medicine
- Medical Genetics
- Neurological Surgery
- Nuclear Medicine
- Obstetrics and Gynecology
- Ophthalmology
- Orthopaedic Surgery
- Otolaryngology
- Pathology
- Pediatrics
- Physical Medicine and Rehabilitation
- Plastic Surgery
- Preventive Medicine
- Psychiatry and Neurology
- Radiology
- Surgery
- Thoracic Surgery
- Urology

19.7 National Residency Matching Program (NRMP)

The National Resident Matching Program (NRMP) (or the Match) is a United States-based private nonprofit nongovernmental organization created in 1952 to help match medical school students with residency programs. The NRMP is sponsored by the American Board of Medical Specialties (ABMS), the American Medical Association (AMA), the Association of American Medical Colleges (AAMC), the

American Hospital Association (AHA), and the Council of Medical Specialty Societies (CMSS).

Virtually every medical student seeking a residency position will enter into The Match. Your schools will train and assist you for this process. To date, it is the fairest system in which you will rank your choices, and the residency programs will rank their choices. A computer will then generate a rank list which will tell you where you are going to train. The process is quite innovative and detailed, and fair.

19.8   Educational Council for Foreign Medical Graduates

The ECFMG is a world leader in promoting quality health care—serving physicians, members of the medical education and regulatory communities, healthcare consumers, and those researching issues in medical education and health workforce planning.

International medical graduates (IMGs) comprise one-quarter of the U.S. physician workforce. Certification by ECFMG is the standard for evaluating the qualifications of these physicians before they enter U.S. graduate medical education (GME), where they provide supervised patient care. ECFMG Certification also is a requirement for IMGs to take Step 3 of the United States Medical Licensing Examination (USMLE) and to obtain an unrestricted license to practice medicine in the United States.

The ECFMG provides other programs for IMGs pursuing U.S. GME, including those that assist them with the process of applying for U.S. GME positions and that sponsor foreign nationals for the J-1 visa for the purpose of participating in such programs. The ECFMG offers a verification service that allows GME programs, state medical boards, hospitals, and credentialing agencies in the United States to obtain primary-source confirmation that their IMG applicants are certified by ECFMG.

The ECFMG partners with the National Board of Medical Examiners (NBME) in administering the Step 2 Clinical Skills (CS) component of USMLE, a requirement for IMGs and for graduates of U.S. and Canadian medical schools who wish to be licensed in the United States or Canada. Through this collaboration, ECFMG uses its experience in assessment to ensure that all physicians entering U.S. GME can demonstrate the fundamental clinical skills essential to providing safe and effective patient care under supervision.

Chapter 20
The Boards

Perhaps the most valuable result of all education is the ability to make yourself do the thing you have to do, when it ought to be done, whether you like it or not; it is the first lesson that ought to be learned; and however early a man's training begins, it is probably the last lesson that he learns thoroughly.

—Thomas H. Huxley (1825–1895)

Preparation for eventual board certification begins the day you start your training, regardless of specialty. The Board certification process is composed of three parts: a written examination, an oral examination, and some kind of case log. The written exam is fairly straightforward. Throughout your training, and after, you will systematically study all of the disciplines and take a multiple choice test. If you pass, you will be permitted to take the oral exam, which will not only test your knowledge, but will actually test your personal skills by demonstrating to the examiner(s) that you are the kind of person who will be safe enough to be considered board certified.

L.D. Florman, *The Portable Medical Mentor: Training Success*, DOI 10.1007/978-3-319-09852-4_20, © Springer International Publishing Switzerland 2015

20.1   The In-Service Exam

Most specialties offer an in-service examination. This provides the program director an opportunity for an annual evaluation of the core curriculum. Your performance will be compared to that of all other residents in the country, in your specialty, in your year of training. This record will become a part of your permanent resident file and could be a deciding factor in determining whether you advance to the senior year, as well as whether you graduate. The examination scores may be included in any letter of recommendation/support for future employment, as well as for sitting for the boards.

You can see that constant preparation is necessary. If your training program has a course of study for the exam, don't miss a single session. If it does not, you should organize your colleagues and systematically tackle every discipline, the so-called core curriculum that will be on the exam. Constantly review the basic sciences. Keep up to date on current readings. Read everything you can put your hands on. Study for this examination as you will eventually study for the Boards. It's your job.

20.2   Tips for Remembering and Studying for Tests

We should not be pretentious enough to teach you how to study. After all, you have, or will graduate from medical school, and that was no easy task. Nonetheless, read these tips on studying and perhaps you will gain some new ideas.

- It is important to form strong impressions of things you wish to remember with as much detail as possible, but separate the wheat from the chaff.
- Study with the intention of remembering by mentally repeating or by writing the item.
- Try to do something with the information you have learned as soon as possible.

- Try to associate a new fact with something that you already know.
- Review what you have learned previously a few days after you reviewed the material for the first time.
- Try to learn material as a whole instead of isolated, separate parts so that it fits into context.
- When studying one subject and switching to another, take a brief rest. When changing subjects, try to go to a topic that is entirely different after the break.
- Have confidence in your memory and your ability to retain information.
- Don't skip classes or assigned reading material.
- Stay awake. Sit in front of the room. Whatever it takes, be aware and stay focused.
- Stay focused on the topic. Don't let your mind wonder by daydreaming about another subject.
- Realize that success on a test is similar to the success in patient care. Both will give you pleasure.
- When studying, it may be necessary to read aloud to keep on subject.
- Know definitions. Don't use terms unless you understand and know the definition of the terminology.
- Stay alert. Turn off your TV. CONCENTRATE.

Chapter 21
The 80-h Week

"Sometimes it is not enough to do our best; we must do what is required."

—Sir Winston Churchill

21.1 Duty Hours Policy for Third and Fourth Years

Duty hours are defined as all clinical and academic activities related to the rotation, i.e., patient care (both inpatient and outpatient), out-of-hospital/clinic time spent on patient notes, administrative duties related to patient care, time spent in-house during shift activities, and scheduled activities, such as conferences.

- Duty hours must be limited to 80 h per week, inclusive of all direct patient care activities (whether completed in-house or at home). Such activities may include writing patient notes and research specifically aimed at writing those notes, as well as preparing to present during daily rounds. Duty hours also include didactic teaching sessions. Duty hours do *not* include time spent studying for exams or for preparation for formal presentations (such as journal clubs, handout development).

L.D. Florman, *The Portable Medical Mentor:*
Training Success, DOI 10.1007/978-3-319-09852-4_21,
© Springer International Publishing Switzerland 2015

- Medical students must be provided with 24 h off after every 7 days of duty, averaged over 4 weeks, free from all educational and clinical responsibilities.
- Continuous on-site duty, including in-house call, must not exceed 24 consecutive hours per day for patient care, plus 4 additional hours for educational activities (e.g., transition of care, conferences).
- At-home call must not be so frequent as to preclude rest and reasonable personal time for each student. When the student is called into the hospital, the hours spent in-house are counted towards the 80-h limit.
- Night float rotation should not exceed six nights in a row; at a minimum there are 8 h off between shifts.
- The student duty hour guidelines will be communicated to students and supervising physicians (including residents, fellows, and faculty) in writing as well as to students verbally during their Transitional Clerkship and at each clerkship orientation.
- Duty hours will be monitored at the end of the block through Evalue; if a student is concerned about a violation of the duty hours policy at a site, the student can fill out an "on-the-fly" report which will go to the Clerkship Director anonymous.

21.2   Duty Hours Policy for Residents and Fellows

- The maximum shift length is 30 h, with 5-h protected sleep time between required shifts, or a maximum of 16 h without protected sleep time.
- The maximum frequency of in-hospital call is every third night.
- The minimum time off between scheduled shifts is 10 h after a day shift, 12 h after a night shift, and 14 h after any extended duty of 30 h [and residents should not return to service earlier than 6 a.m. the next day].

- The maximum frequency of in-hospital night shifts is four nights sequentially. After three or four night shifts, a student must have at least 48 continuous hours off before the next shift.
- As a minimum, a student must have the following days off duty: 5 days per month, 1 day (24 h) per week, and one continuous 48-h period off per month.
- In exceptional circumstances, the time on duty can be increased to 88 h for select programs with a sound educational rationale.
- In the emergency department, the maximum shift limit is 12 h, with at least an equivalent time between shifts. The maximum number of shift hours per week is 60 h, with an additional 12 h permitted for education.

The educational goals of residency training programs and the learning objectives of residents must not be compromised by excessive clinical service obligations. The Accreditation Council on Graduate Medical Education (ACGME) has charged sponsoring institutions with ensuring that formal written policies governing resident duty hours be established at both the institutional and program level.

Each sponsored program must have a formal written policy on resident duty hours. The ACGME regulations are listed below. It should be understood that each program and institution has adapted these rules; however, the minimum requirements apply to all interns, residents, and fellows.

- Duty hours must not exceed 80 h per week averaged over 4 weeks. Duty hours are defined as:
  - All clinical activities relating to the residency program.
  - All academic activities relating to the residency program.
  - All administrative duties relating to the residency program.
  - All patient care duties.
  - All conferences.
  - All on-call time.
  - All moonlighting hours

- Residents must be given 10 h off for rest and personal activities between duty periods and after call.
- In-house call must occur no more frequently than every third night, averaged over 4 weeks.
- Resident assignments must not exceed 24 h maximum, continuous on-site duty, with up to 6 additional hours permitted for patient transfer and other activities defined in RRC requirements.
- A resident must not be assigned new patients after 24 h of continuous duty.
- Resident time spent in the hospital during at-home call must be counted towards the 80 h. At home call is not subject to the every third night limitation.
- "Moonlighting" (spare time work):

  - Must be approved by the program director. Some programs specifically forbid it.
  - Must not interfere with your ability to achieve the goals and objectives of the educational program.
  - Must be monitored to ensure that you comply with the program and institutional policies.
  - Work outside the residency program and the institution does not count against the 80 h.
  - Internal moonlighting (i.e., within the program or institution) must be counted towards the 80-h weekly limit on duty hours.

- All residents must be provided with 1 day in 7 free from all educational and clinical responsibilities, averaged over a 4-week period, inclusive of call. "One day" is defined as one continuous 24-h period.
- Duty hours must be monitored by the program. Most programs will require weekly written reports and a quarterly time study. Some programs satisfy the reporting requirements online.
- Program directors must develop and have in place policies to prevent and counteract the effects of resident fatigue.
- Backup support must be provided when needed.

Always consult the rules specific to your residency training program and hospital. These rules must be taken very seriously because your program could lose its accreditation if they are violated. Some states have statutes concerning these rules, thereby making them the law. If broken, someone could actually be fined or go to jail.

Chapter 22
Research

> "Research is what I'm doing when I don't know what I'm doing."
>
> — Werner Von Braun

Medical doctors are physicians first, and scientists second. The advanced state of modern medicine has been made possible only by the hard work of our always inquisitive forefathers. It is our turn to carry on this very important and ancient tradition of intellectual curiosity, discovery, and inventiveness in medicine. There is no place for complacency in medical thought. It is necessary to keep one's eyes, ears, and mind open to the never-ending river of questions generated by today's practice of the healing arts.

Ideas for research are limited only by one's imagination and perseverance, and this provides the nidus for tomorrow's advancements in every aspect of the practice of medicine. Always be on the lookout for questions that need answers, for disease processes that beg for elucidation and treatment, for instruments that need an operation (or vice versa), and for better and newer ways of doing things.

Don't be hesitant to discuss ideas with your attendings, your colleagues, or the appropriate laboratory people. Jot down your ideas in your little black book so that they are not forgotten. Remember, no idea is too insignificant.

L.D. Florman, *The Portable Medical Mentor:*
Training Success, DOI 10.1007/978-3-319-09852-4_22,
© Springer International Publishing Switzerland 2015

Many residency training programs require 1 year of research or at least one peer reviewed publication. If you are considering a career in academic medicine, research and publishing will be mandatory. If you are a student anticipating one of the high profile residencies (surgery, dermatology, otolaryngology, radiology, etc.), now is the time to get involved with one of the many research activities taking place in your medical school. Interviewers at residency training programs are very impressed with students who have participated in research projects. The same goes for those seeking fellowship positions. Regardless of what stage of your training, get involved. It is not only personally very rewarding, but also, in some little, or large way, serves the cause for the advancement of medicine.

Most university websites list the ongoing research projects by department.

Chapter 23
Interviews

"Sow a thought and you reap an action;
Sow an act and you reap a habit;
Sow a habit and you reap a character;
Sow a character and you reap a destiny."

—Buddhist Proverb

23.1 General

Placement for training positions in the high-profile residencies and fellowships has historically been quite competitive. Today, obtaining one of these sacred residencies or fellowships is more of a challenge when considering their decreasing numbers, the increasing quality and credentials of the applicants, and, in most instances, the rather mechanical nature of the "match." From start to finish of this grueling, complicated, meticulous, and often expensive process the student (or resident) is required to portray his or her life in the best light possible, so as to impress the reviewer(s) to the point where they will ultimately be ranked, and get the job. So many factors in this selection process are, in reality, so completely out of your control that you had at least better increase your chances of acceptance by making an immaculate application and interview.

L.D. Florman, *The Portable Medical Mentor:*
Training Success, DOI 10.1007/978-3-319-09852-4_23,
© Springer International Publishing Switzerland 2015

The essence of this chapter is provided by experienced reviewers who have read thousands of applications, have interviewed hundreds of applicants, and have accepted only a few candidates. These are only a few tips. Remember that once you are granted an interview, the rest of the process is purely up to your performance when meeting face to face with the interviewers. A great interview can make up for certain inadequacies in your application.

23.2   The Preparation

You began to prepare when you entered medical school.

- You made good grades, or the best that you could.
- You tried for honors courses.
- You volunteered for anything and everything.
- You sat in front of the lecture room.
- You worked in a research laboratory.
- You asked good questions.
- You read this book and lived the spirit of it.

    During the clinical years:

- You arrived earlier and left later than your fellow students.
- You worked hard to learn and secondarily to impress your attendings and residents.
- You asked good questions.
- You listened carefully.
- You continued to work in the research laboratory.
- You worked towards getting you name listed on publications.
- You nurtured your relationship with the professor in charge of your research laboratory. Hopefully he or she is going to write a letter of recommendation for you.
- You did not antagonize any secretaries in the department. They are really important. Secretaries "run the world."

- The residents and fellows you rotated with have sterling comments to make about your work. When questioned by an attending, an angry resident can do you a great deal of harm, or good.
- You read this book, and lived the spirit of it.

If you are applying for a residency or fellowship position from a residency or a fellowship position, then your mission becomes more detailed and more competitive.

- Applicants named in several publications look great.
- Applicants with transferable research grants are irresistible.
- You must read this book again and live by the spirit of it.

23.3   The Application

The written application is the easiest part of your documentation. Just do it correctly, neatly, and timely. It is at this time that you might communicate with the secretaries or coordinators of the institutions that you are applying to. Be absolutely professional, courteous, and just plain nice. They often have a "say." You can be sure that if you antagonize one of them, or, in frustration, speak harshly to one of them, it will get back to the chairman, and you will not get the job.

- Type the entire application.
- Do not use initials anywhere on the application.
- Do not be too trite or clichéd in your personal statement.
- Attempt to record your greatest achievements in a moderate fashion. In other words, the reviewers can also read between the lines.

23.4   The Interview

A discussion of this aspect of the application process is the main purpose of this chapter. If the written application is the crown of your achievements, the interview is your personal castle. It is your special time to come out, to shine, to impress, and perhaps to beg a little. Everything must be perfect. However, being perfect is usually not enough. You must be better than all of the other applicants. Your history speaks for itself and is unalterable. Now you have to show the real you.

- Be early for your interview.
- Do you know how to dress?

  For men, dark suit (no pinstripes), subdued but sharp necktie (preferably predominately red), polished shoes, well cut hair and groomed. No jewelry except for a wedding band (if you are married). No watch or bracelet. Facial hair in some programs is frowned upon.

  For women, dark pants suit or dress suit, minimal jewelry, only one small earring in each ear, no high heels, absolutely no cleavage (certain interviewers resent that an applicant may believe that showing a little cleavage or thigh might influence their decision). Actually, it may negatively influence it. Wear something red (a bangle, a necklace).

- Often, secretaries, coordinators, interns, and residents will be around to assist in the interview process. Get close to them. Talk to them. Be nice to them. Don't ask them any stupid questions (like "Is there a workout room in the hospital?"). They will be asked for their opinion about you. And, their opinion really matters.
- Shake hands solidly, not like a wet fish.
- Do not fidget.
- Sit up straight on the edge of your chair.
- Address each interviewer by their name. Never look at the ceiling, the floor, the table, or into space. Make eye contact all the time.
- Never say "yeh." Always say "yes sir, no sir (or mam)." Never say "you know!" or "you know?" Do not say "I probably …." Say "I definitely …" or "I immediately …." Sound like you mean it.
- Never say "well, to tell you the truth …," or "honestly." You better be telling the truth.

- Never say "Oh, that's a good question." They will be thinking that of course it is a good question or I wouldn't have asked it.
- Answer all questions without beating around the bush. Be direct, forceful, assertive, and certain. Make sure that you answer questions in the context that they are asked.
- Smile
- Don't embellish too much. Certainly don't brag.
- The idea is to get the interviewer to like you and trust you. All of the details of your life are on the written application. The interview makes it all personal, and helps fill in the spaces between the words.
- Demonstrate your compassion and your ability to work hard.
- Make the interviewer want to be with you for the next few years. He will be able to tell in a few short minutes that you are the kind of person who will be a pleasure to teach.
- Most likely there will not be any medical questions. But if there are, the reason will probably be to see the process that you use to address them, rather than the final answer.
- Read this book again.

Some schools have faculty members who give mock interviews. If you have the opportunity to do this, by all means take advantage of it.

23.5 The Match

Many candidates for residency and fellowship positions will be applying through the National Residency Matching Program (NRMP), commonly called "the match," the details of which are beyond the scope of this book. The match is a sort of computer game which at a point in the process, takes out the humanism, and relegates your future to a computer program. Actually it is most likely the fairest way to deal with so many applications.

Do not violate any of the match rules or dates.

23.6   Away Rotations

If your school permits away rotations in the third or fourth year, and if you are fairly sure of your specialty choice, then an away rotation can be very advantageous to you. Consider the away rotation as a month-long interview. Be sure to take advantage of a mock interview prior to the rotation if your school offers them. If your school does not offer them, then ask an instructor to put one together for you.

During the away rotation try and warm up to the program director and the chairman of the department. Ingratiate yourself to all of the residents, but don't get too chummy with them. Ultimately, they will be asked about you. Don't vocalize your desire for an ultimate subspecialty. No program director wants a first-year resident who is aiming for one of the subspecialties. And, the residents will talk. Remember that each resident that you contact has a friend who will ultimately vie for the position that you are applying for.

Of course, away rotations are great for you to carefully inspect the program and the residents. Is this the place where you want to spend the next few years of your training? Are the residents happy? Is the patient variety ample and varied?

Chapter 24
HIPAA

If you reveal your secrets to the wind, you should
not blame the wind for revealing them to the trees.

— Khalil Gibran

The *Health Insurance Portability and Accountability Act of
1996 (HIPAA)* was instituted in the USA to ensure the protection of individuals' health information while also allowing
communication between parties involved with patient care.
It was not until 1999, however, when the US Department of
Health and Human Services developed the Privacy Rule that
made implementation of HIPAA mandatory. Effective from
April 2003, organizations (i.e., "covered entities") subject to
HIPAA regulations were required to comply with patient
information protection policies. "Covered entities" refer to
health plans, healthcare providers, and healthcare clearing-
houses. HIPAA rules are constantly being modified, the last
significant change having taken place at the beginning of 2014.

Required disclosures of identifiable individual health
information include a request by a patient for his/her information or a request by the US Department of Health and

L.D. Florman, *The Portable Medical Mentor:*
Training Success, DOI 10.1007/978-3-319-09852-4_24,
© Springer International Publishing Switzerland 2015

Human Services in special instances, such as a review. The privacy rule outlines six permitted disclosures of individual health information, including the following:

- Per request of the patient.
- For treatment, payment, and healthcare operations.
- To individuals identified by the patient, who may be informed; in emergency situations, the healthcare provider must use his/her professional judgment to determine the best interest of the patient.
- Incidental disclosure.
- Limited data set with the removal of certain individual identifiers.
- Public interest, which encompasses disclosures required by law; public health activities; abuse, neglect, and domestic violence; health oversight activities; judicial and administrative proceedings; law enforcement purposes; decedents; cadaver organ and tissue donation; research with permission of governing body, such as Institutional Review Board; threat to health or society; essential government functions; worker compensation.

State governments reserve the right to have supplemental policies to further increase patient privacy protection. Check with your institution to determine additional policies and guidelines.

In short, treat identifiable health information as patient property. Be careful how, where, and to whom you discuss and distribute patient information. Protection of patient privacy rights is required by law.

Suggestions for HIPAA Compliance

- Be aware of your surroundings.
- Do not discuss patients in public places such as elevators, waiting rooms, public hallways, and lobbies.
- Dispose of identifiable health information, such as patient lists, in the appropriate manner. Most hospitals have labeled containers for material that is to be shredded.

- Do not publicly display patient information. This includes both in hospitals and outpatient clinics (i.e., do not leave patient charts unattended, or on computer monitors).
- When discussing scenarios or presenting a case to individuals not directly involved in the care of a patient, do not disclose identifiable patient information.
- Do not identify patients over the Internet.

24.1   HIPAA at a Glance

24.1.1   What Is HIPAA?

- Governs the use and disclosure of protected health information (PHI) that is created or received by a covered entity that relates to:

  - The physical or mental health of an individual (living or deceased).
  - The provision of health care.
  - The payment for health care.
  - Identifies the individual or reasonably may be used to identify the individual.

- Gives individuals the following rights. The right to …

  - Request restrictions on use or disclosure of their personal health information.
  - Access medical records (including research records).
  - Amend medical records.
  - An accounting of disclosure of their personal health information.
  - Request alternate confidential communications.
  - Lodge complaint with covered entity and/or the Department for Health and Human Services.

- Administrative requirements. The covered entity must …

  - Designate a privacy official.
  - Develop policies and procedures that are HIPAA compliant.
  - Provide privacy training to the workforce.

– Implement administrative, technical, and physical safeguards to protect the privacy of personal health information.
– Develop sanctions for violations of the HIPAA Privacy Rule.
– Meet the documentation requirements.

• Enforcement/penalties (individual, not institutional).

– Civil penalties:

  (a) $100 for each violation, up to $25,000/person/year.
  (b) Liability exists if a person knew, or reasonably should have known, of a violation and did not try to rectify the situation.

– Criminal penalties:

  (a) Knowing:

    Up to $50,000/year and/or imprisonment of up to 1 year.

  (b) False pretenses:

    Up to $100,000/year and/or imprisonment of up to 5 years.

  (c) Intent to sell, transfer, or use for commercial advantage, personal gain, or malicious harm.

    Up to $250,000/year and/or imprisonment of up to 10 years.

• Impact on researchers

– Recruitment of subjects
– If a subject refuses to authorize the use and disclosure of public health information, the individual cannot participate in the research study.
– Accounting for disclosures:

  (a) Preparatory to research.
  (b) Waiver of authorization.
  (c) Decedent data.

- Allowable uses and disclosures of PHI for research.
  - Authorization from subject.
  - Waiver of authorization from IRB.
  - Use of de-identified data.
  - Use of limited data set.
  - Preparatory to research.
  - Decedent data.

It is obvious that HIPAA has necessitated a whole new nomenclature for physicians, all individuals in the healthcare industry, and certainly for the patients who are protected by it. Interestingly, HIPAA is nothing new to physicians. In 400 B.C.E. Hippocrates, acclaimed as the father of medicine, proclaimed in his oath that we should uphold the privacy of our patients. This is also addressed in the modern version of the *Hippocratic Oath*.

24.2   Hippocratic Oath: Classic Version

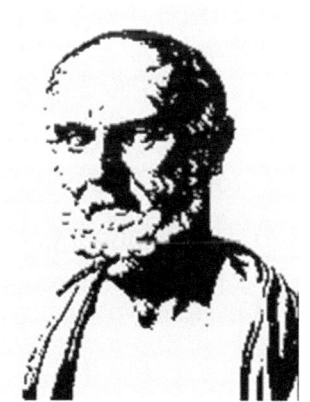

FIG. 24.1. Hippocrates of Kos (19th century engraving, artist unknown)

I swear by Apollo Physician and Asclepius and Hygieia and Panaceia and all the gods and goddesses, making them my witnesses, that I will fulfill according to my ability and judgment this oath and this covenant:

To hold him who has taught me this art as equal to my parents and to live my life in partnership with him, and if he is in need of money to give him a share of mine, and to regard his offspring as equal to my brothers in male lineage and to teach them this art—if they desire to learn it—without fee and covenant; to give a share of precepts and oral instruction and all the other learning to my sons and to the sons of him who has instructed me and to pupils who have signed the covenant and have taken an oath according to the medical law, but no one else.

I will apply dietetic measures for the benefit of the sick according to my ability and judgment; I will keep them from harm and injustice.

I will neither give a deadly drug to anybody who asked for it, nor will I make a suggestion to this effect. Similarly I will not give to a woman an abortive remedy. In purity and holiness I will guard my life and my art.

I will not use the knife, not even on sufferers from stone, but will withdraw in favor of such men as are engaged in this work.

Whatever houses I may visit, I will come for the benefit of the sick, remaining free of all intentional injustice, of all mischief and in particular of sexual relations with both female and male persons, be they free or slaves.

What I may see or hear in the course of the treatment or even outside of the treatment in regard to the life of men, which on no account one must spread abroad, I will keep to myself, holding such things shameful to be spoken about.

If I fulfill this oath and do not violate it, may it be granted to me to enjoy life and art, being honored with fame among all men for all time to come; if I transgress it and swear falsely, may the opposite of all this be my lot.

Chapter 25
Social Media

25.1 Introduction

Social media refers to a relatively new development in communications. From large, well-known media sites to smaller, boutique websites social media dominates the future of communication in the twenty-first century. The content of this form of media is entirely user generated. It is deemed "social" as early forms of this medium were based on established connections from non-digital arenas and the majority of the interactions on these media formats take the form of social interactions instead of professional interactions or monetary transactions.

Social media has revolutionized the way people communicate directly, and about ideas. The instantaneous flow of communication across social networks in the digital medium has made the world a much smaller place than ever before. It is now not only possible, but also easy for a person experiencing violence and oppression in the third world to leverage these Web-based platforms into social actions. On the flip side, it has also never been easier to share a video of your cat or force others to ogle pictures of your dessert creation.

In recent years, social media has combined those real-life connections with virtual ones, allowing people with similar interests and views to express themselves in a single community

L.D. Florman, *The Portable Medical Mentor:*
Training Success, DOI 10.1007/978-3-319-09852-4_25,
© Springer International Publishing Switzerland 2015

even though they may be separated over vast distances. Over the past few years, varying forms of social media have developed. Social media was among the factors precipitating the Arab Spring, allowing for the notable revolutions in Libya and Egypt, as well as other locations.

Like any form of media, social media has its stars and those trying to use this media form as a way to make a name for themselves. Some leverage the power of social media to produce content that will generate advertising revenue. Others use it as a form of hard-sell self-promotion. Many organizations will use it as a platform for distributing the message they espouse.

Your role as a training physician is to understand the:

1. Various forms of social media and how they relate both to your personal life and career.
2. Advantages that social media can grant you.
3. Disadvantages that social media may foist upon you.
4. Special considerations you must think of as a professional, not just a physician.

25.2   Specific Examples of Social Media

25.2.1   Facebook

Infamously founded by the Harvard Educated Mark Zuckerburg and now the largest social network at play in America, Facebook is by now a common part of your vocabulary as house officer. Many young people do not remember a time in their social lives when Facebook was not a part of it. Attempting to qualify Facebook as a social media is difficult. It facilitates interaction between those you know and those you don't. It allows for personal endorsement of not just products, but companies, organizations, and even abstract concepts such as "cancer screening."

Facebook goes beyond endorsement and "likes." It allows users to post virtually any information they would like about themselves. Pictures are a frequent post, especially of social events. Companies use Facebook as a mechanism to promote products and conducts giveaways that were formally the purview of packaging or television advertising campaigns.

Previously popular with teens as a way to post information, trade messages, and have conversations, Facebook has seen a massive decline in users between the age of 13 and 25 over the past 3 years. The user base of Facebook has now shifted essentially to those of Generation X and older. Facebook was the first social media site to undergo an IPO on the stock market, as well.

Physicians most typically use Facebook as a means to either (1) promote their practice/hospital or (2) endorse causes. A prime example would be physician endorsements and reposts of messages from the Susan G. Komen foundation. Physicians rarely use Facebook as a portal of communication with patients as the messages through this service are not secure. Though the Affordable Care Act requires the ability of each physician to communicate with patients via a secure web portal, Facebook is not the correct mechanism.

25.2.2   Twitter

140 characters doesn't seem like much. However, when you add in the ability to direct them to specific people with "@" and promote ideas with "#" (aka the "hashtag") you get a social platform that has been wildly successful. Twitter has become extremely popular over the past few years, largely supplanting Facebook as the social media vehicle of choice for people under the age of 25–30. Twitter allows for the posting of text of less than 140 characters, private messages, photos, and videos of less than 6 s (called "Vines"). Links are often a frequent post as well. Each of these messages is called a "Tweet."

Twitter serves as a point of entry from fans to celebrities. A user can "follow" the account of a specific celebrity, colleague, or organization. This results in message sent to their own account whenever those they follow provide an update. The use of smartphone technology has propagated this further as the ability to "push" notifications about Twitter allows for frequent, mobile updates. Indeed, updates to twitter can occur via simple text message using SMS protocol.

The simplicity and mobility of the platform are its strength. This allows for virtually anyone with a cell phone and an account to post to Twitter anywhere there is cell phone service. This facility is what aided the Libyan rebels in coordinating and launching a successful revolution against the Gaddafi regime.

Physicians so far have used Twitter in a variety of ways. Using sponsored posts (read: "advertisements") to promote a particular procedure, clinic, or field of expertise. Large physician organizations also will have Twitter accounts to disseminate useful links and upcoming initiatives. The American College of Surgeons has a reliable Twitter feed for updates on happenings in surgery across the country. Physicians also have used Twitter as a way to keep up with professional societies and groups of particular subspecialty interest. A search for potential Twitter accounts to follow depending on your interest in various fields is below. The list is very short. Most societies are still breaking into this market with very few having true social media campaigns. This area is ripe for development for an entrepreneurial, tech-savvy surgeon to help out the leadership of these organizations.

25.2.3   LinkedIn

LinkedIn purports to be the professional answer to Facebook. Using LinkedIn, a user can post a resume, highlight professional connections, and post job skills. The unique aspect of LinkedIn is the "endorsement system." A user's contacts and "connections" can endorse the user for various skills that they display on their digital profile or resume. Connections are also free to add other endorsements that the user may not have thought of, thereby growing the online professional profile of the user. Some companies will have a LinkedIn profile, but it is mostly for individuals. More employers are asking for LinkedIn profiles during interviews. It will likely not come up during a residency or fellowship interview, but it is increasingly more common for employers to expect this during the actual job search. This is doubly true at major academic universities and large corporate health systems.

25.2.4 Photoblogs

Several different versions of photoblogs have appeared over the past few years, each with its own particular tweak on the way that users share photos with other users.

Instagram's popularity has soared in the past 2 years. Users of Instagram typically use an application on a mobile device to take photos and upload them to Instagram with certain hashtags (#) for identification by other users.

Pinterest is similar, but instead of uploading original photos, users "pin" or virtually collect pictures and associated articles to a virtual pinboard allowing for later reference. This simultaneously creates a cross section of the users' interests and likes. (This is a BRILLIANT scheme, as they can charge a fortune for truly directed advertising, expecting a better return on niche markets for every marketing dollar spent).

Tumblr is a partial photo-blogging vs. blogging site that is where the more unseemly portion of the Internet can bleed through into social media. The vast majority of users, however, simply use Tumblr as an online diary of sorts with an attached comment section for interaction with other users.

25.2.5 Google +

Though currently listed as the number five overall social network in terms of discrete hits in March 2014, Google+ has yet to truly catch on in many American circles. Its use has replaced the previously used Google Talk Web-based VOIP service to a large degree. Specific features include the ability to group contacts into "circles" such as "family" and "work". In addition, Google hangouts provide users the ability to have a static video chat online that is available to anyone they approve. This is an attractive thought for example, for a physician. If you wanted to establish some form of "virtual office hours" where patients could call you with questions via a professional Google account, they could contact you at any time when you are completing charts in your office or other tasks, simply by having the appropriate Hangout open and available.

25.2.6 *YouTube*

The 1,000 lb gorilla in the room of the media landscape for the near future is YouTube. What was once a collection of funny home movies and relatively everyday videos has grown immensely. There are entire features produced exclusively for YouTube consumption. Virtually every TV set made today has YouTube built in as an "app." The content on YouTube is becoming more complex daily with dedicated channels for each type of content. YouTube is the number one way that people under the age of 20 consume music via streaming the video. Interestingly, YouTube has brought about the return of the 30-s commercial to the Internet video industry, and many video producers are living entirely off of the revenue generated by these ads.

Physicians have been more active on YouTube than other forms of social media. Typically videos of physicians have been profiled so that potential patients may learn more about them, technique videos for surgeons, or educational videos for patients about a particular topic. While there are many of these videos available, they are usually of middling quality. This is a potential area of improvement for a young physician with the appropriate skills.

25.3   Advantages/Possibilities with Social Media

The ability of social media to supplement your professional appearance cannot be understated. As patients take more and more to the Internet and their mobile devices for information, it would behoove each physician to develop a strong, and consistent online presence. This means that whichever avenues of social media you pursue, you need to be consistent across them. Having a clear, cogent message to portray across all platforms will allow those finding you on more than one platform to understand your clinical goals.

Additionally, having a social media presence will allow you to have Internet referral metrics. Social media sites have dedicated metrics in place that show users the number of "hits" they have gotten, as well as the number of each user's proprietary measurement of success. For example, Twitter can show user the number of followers they have. This information can be further mined to determine when the followers accessed your account most recently, how long they followed you, what other accounts they follow, and the number of times they have accessed your account to read your posts. When grouped together across platforms, these access metrics can provide information as to whether your particular message is working or is falling upon deaf screens/mice.

25.4   Disadvantages in Social Media

It cannot be said enough times that posting on social media as a professional trying to market yourself to patients is dangerous business. Simple things such as family photos pose little professional liability. However, the posting of your wild weekend in Cabo can be very deleterious to your career. Keep your personal life away from the view of the public using the various settings available to you through each website, and be thoughtful in your personal posts. Avoid posting anything that might embarrass your grandmother, and consider going back to clean up your current social media accounts. Create a separate business account for your practice and one for home/personal use with limited access. This will serve as a portal for your patients and keep separate your business and personal contacts as well.

Social media as an endeavor is a task with momentum. In order to maintain that momentum, if you post weekly you will lose followers and interest if you don't continue that trend. That is true even if the post is minimal. The most successful people on social media are those that understand their audience, speak directly to their audience, and do so frequently. If you are going to start a social media campaign, make sure that you follow through.

Be sure to source other people's materials properly, even though social media is a casual format. The rules of intellectual property still apply. Don't get caught with your pants down by the uncredited use of an image or webpage. Your own material should be similarly copy written.

25.5   Special Comment: HIPAA

HIPPA applies to online posts just as any other forum. The temptation to take photos of potentially horrible things or interesting findings on call and then post them to social media sites will be omnipresent, but you must resist. Most healthcare organizations strictly forbid this, and it will likely result in your being fired. The same is true of communications about specific patients and their health. All the laws of HIPAA apply to the patient's information whether physical or virtual. Be careful what you post about your job and make sure not to give any identifying information over the Internet.

Chapter 26
Electronic Medical Record

A component of recent medical legislation has been the institution of the electronic medical record (EMR) for all healthcare systems by the end of calendar 2014. That said, the EMR can take any number of forms. Some EMRs are simply a compilation of scanned paper charts. Others are entirely electronic with all note entry, order entry, image reporting, prescribing, and billing occurring with a contained single program. These programs are the future portal of your daily routine in health care so understanding how the record in your particular system works is not only essential to your workflow as a resident or fellow, but also necessary to the student to be able to glean records and lab results for patients on their service. The ins and outs of each EMR is beyond the scope of this book; however, here we discuss a few pointers to using the electronic medical record in your care of patients, and things to avoid.

There is a strong learning curve with the EMR, and most hospitals have their own system which usually requires some kind of intensive indoctrination in the form of mandatory instruction.

L.D. Florman, *The Portable Medical Mentor:*
Training Success, DOI 10.1007/978-3-319-09852-4_26,
© Springer International Publishing Switzerland 2015

26.1   Helpful Pointers for Using the EMR as a Resident: How to Look Put Together on Morning Rounds

– As soon as you get to the hospital print out a patient list to carry with you; trying to drag an iPad or similar device to each patients room every morning when you are trying to get rounds done quickly will slow you down as you try to look up results, consultations, progress notes, etc. Save the iPad for rounds with your chief/attending.

– Make notes on your list of pertinent findings in the EMR. Do not write down the vital signs, labs, or intake/output until you have more time. You can fill these in using the EMR on your electronic notepad.

– See the patients—take quick, but careful notes. Don't write a progress note until all patients have been seen.

– Once your team has seen all patients, sit down and write your notes based on all the data you have amassed from your early AM computer sweep, RN notes, exam that morning, and now labs/vitals/radiographic results.

– Once your notes are in—make it a point to recheck the EMR at certain scheduled times during the day. Changes will be made, attendings will write notes behind you, and plans will be updated. If your attending plans to get a CT and you beat him/her to the order because you saw it in their note you look like a star. Attendings love it when you say, "I read your note and the response from the ICU attending, I think we should pursue course X because,…" Then you, of course, go on to quote some esoteric but brilliant piece of medical literature and win all the resident awards for your program.

26.2 Potential Pitfalls for the EMR: How to Look Like You Don't Know What You Are Doing

- Don't write notes after seeing each patient in the morning, you will get behind!
- Only document what you actually did; it is easy to get in the habit of checking off on "a full 12 point review of systems was performed" or "Regular Rate/Rhythm, normal S1/S2, no edema" when you didn't actually do a ROS or examine a patient's heart. Not only does this provide false information about the patient to other doctors and healthcare professionals, but if you then charge for your erroneous "clicks" you have committed insurance fraud. You can get yourself and your attendings in a bunch of hot water this way, including loss of licensure and major fines. DON'T DO IT! JUST DOCUMENT WHAT YOU DID. If that only amounts to a low/noncomplex billing code, then submit that and move on.
- Don't get frustrated and give up on the EMR. The EMR is here to stay and you must learn how to mine it for information. Take a "super-user" class if you need to. Study about your patients over the net when you get home at night through the web portal of the hospital. There are becoming fewer and fewer excuses for not knowing the pertinent facts of patient care.

Chapter 27
Insurance, Managed Care

27.1   Health Insurance

At the time of this writing the system of healthcare insurance in the United States is undergoing major changes. This changing scenario will likely last for years and will not be pleasant to understand or deal with. You must become at least superficially knowledgeable with the system as it will affect your day to day practice even as a resident or fellow.

Currently, the main mechanism through which health care is administered in the United States comes through health insurance "carried" by patients. At its most basic, insurance allows payment into a group account with later withdrawal based on medical need. This allows for reimbursement to healthcare providers and healthcare organizations as the individual requires care.

Health insurance can take many forms, but the purpose is always the same—provide payment for rendered care. The purpose of this section is to orient you to the various forms of insurance, their meaning for you and your patients, and ultimately how they will affect your care as a medical student/resident. This is by no means a comprehensive list or explanation of the U.S. healthcare system. The easiest way to think of a potential patient's health insurance is to compare groups of insurance providers (Fig. 27.1) and understand their purpose.

L.D. Florman, *The Portable Medical Mentor: Training Success*, DOI 10.1007/978-3-319-09852-4_27,
© Springer International Publishing Switzerland 2015

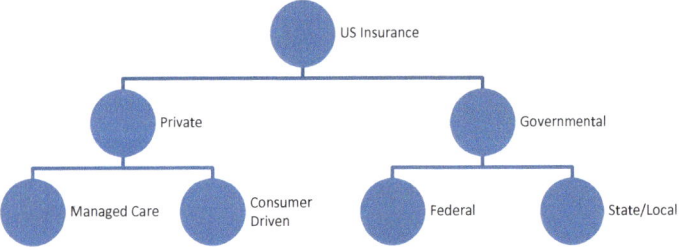

FIG. 27.1. Groups of insurance providers

27.1.1 Private Health Insurance

Private insurance in the U.S. is the most common form you will encounter in the non-elderly. The early part of the twentieth century was dominated by the development of Blue Cross/Blue Shield—a program where doctors and hospitals asked essentially for no copayment (fee at the time of service). They practiced independent of significant oversight. With the advent of Medicare and Medicaid, this changed significantly as the U.S. government was now the largest consumer of health care in the country. Over the latter half of the century, efforts made to control unnecessary spending have led to the forms of insurance we currently have. Specific goals were made in order to prevent unnecessary expenditures, while still maintaining high quality health care.

These forces have led to the development of Managed Care—a powerful force in American health care that you will encounter on a daily basis. In short, managed care organizations are "Health insurance plans intended to reduce unnecessary healthcare costs through a variety of mechanisms." Know that managed care serves as a way to steer healthcare consumers—sometimes in ways you don't intend. While the ideal of Managed Care was designed to allow for oversight of care by the largest consumers of care—large companies—it propagated the concept of mandating specific care patterns. Certain measures are now expected by insurance providers;

TABLE 27.1. List of CMS Never Events

- Pressure ulcer stages III and IV
- Falls and trauma
- Surgical site infection after bariatric surgery for obesity, certain orthopedic procedures, and bypass surgery (mediastinitis)
- Vascular-catheter associated infection
- Catheter-associated urinary tract infection
- Administration of incompatible blood
- Air embolism
- Foreign object unintentionally retained after surgery

others are banned, to the point of non-reimbursement for care should these guidelines not be followed. One of your tasks is to know common guidelines for patient care in your specialty. These are typically established practice parameters that take their cues from sources such as NSQIP (National Surgery Quality Improvement Program) or the list of CMS Never Events (Table 27.1).

Managed Care Organizations usually have a preferred set of providers and coverage "network" they will reimburse. As a student or house officer, being able to understand the varying types of managed care that your patients will have is the most important point. The difficulty becomes in learning the alphabet soup of options that patients will have when they see you. Don't be afraid to look up answers with your patient. It shows that you are in the same boat as they are in navigating the confusing mess that the insurance system has become. Also, if you take the time to help them understand what they are choosing between, you will likely learn more yourself.

The following table (Table 27.2) is meant to serve as a ready reference so that when a patient asks a question about insurance, you can understand what they are saying. The specific options available to patients will change based on where you are practicing, what plans are given through their work, and the patient's income.

Consumer Driven Healthcare is a contemporary invention that developed in response to patients feeling limited in their choices by HMOs and PPOs. Frequently, this type of insurance

TABLE 27.2. Types of Managed Care

Type of insurance	Description
Health Maintenance Organization (HMO)	**An organization of healthcare providers that attempts to service all healthcare needs of a patient within one group** – Coined the term "PCP" to act as a "medical gatekeeper" to referrals to specialists, as well as nonemergent hospital admissions – Usually provided at the corporate level – Must be offered to employees at companies of 25 or more people
Independent Practice Association (IPA)	**A group of physicians that have partnered to improve both quality of patient care and their own bargaining ability** – Accept typical fee-for-service patients – Contract with major insurance corps. or managed care organization to provide care
Preferred Provider Organization (PPO)	**A subset of managed care that contracts with physicians, hospitals, and other entities to provide care at a reduced cost in return for exclusivity** – Can lead to significant cost savings for all involved – Decreases choice of healthcare consumer
Point of Service Plan (POS)	**A plan designed to compromise between the limitation of choice and financial burden of care** – Patients have a preferred network of providers – May move outside that network for a progressively higher fee dependent on the type of service
Private Fee for Service (PFFS)	**Alternative to Managed Care** – **Basic Coverage = most simple form of coverage available. Covers only acute care issues** – **Major Medical Coverage = covers all forms of illness, usually has long-term care component**

takes the form of a given pool of funds given to a patient over the course of year. This pool of funds is intended to pay for all portions of a patient's health: over-the-counter medications, physician copays, and virtually any health expenditure. Once this pool of funds has been depleted, then it functions similar to traditional Fee-For-Service insurance plans. The most common form of this type of insurance is the **Flexible Spending Account (FSA)**.

27.1.2   Governmental Health Insurance

The largest payer within the U.S. healthcare system is the Federal Government. This is a relatively recent event beginning with the advent of Medicare and Medicaid in 1965. Currently, CMS (the Center for Medicare and Medicaid Services) insures roughly one-third of all Americans. The Affordable Care Act (ACA) is projected to expand this by offering coverage to the roughly 41.3 million uninsured Americans. Important to know as well, the vast majority of resident slots in the American system are directly funded by a reimbursement to each individual educational institution.

The most useful thing a young physician can do is to familiarize themselves with the different parts of Medicare/Medicaid and how they will affect the patients that you treat.

Medicare is governmental insurance available to the following groups of people:

- People 65 or older
- People 65 or younger with certain disabilities
- Anyone with End-Stage Renal Disease (ESRD)
- Anyone with Amyotrophic Lateral Sclerosis (ALS)

There are four major components to Medicare, Parts A–D.

- Part A: Hospital Insurance—coverage for admission to a hospital, skilled nursing facility, hospice care, or home health care; usually no charge as long as patient or spouse contributed to Medicare while working.
- Part B: Medical Insurance—services from healthcare providers, outpatient care, home health care, durable medical equipment, some preventive services; this requires a monthly premium, but there may be gaps in the coverage that require filling with a Medigap policy, depending on the amount of coverage desired.
- Part C: Medicare Advantage—run by Medicare approved companies that bundle all components of Medicare with potential for other services as well, likely increased cost over baseline coverage of Parts A/B/D together.

– Part D: Medicare Prescription Drug Coverage—designed to allow for private insurers to provide prescription drug insurance, allows for decreased cost due to larger volume consumption, usually saves patients money in the long term.

Some patients may call upon you to help them decide which form of insurance to choose. While attempting to be helpful, this can easily become more confusing to you both. The best advice you can give patients is a simple primer to the parts of Medicare and encourage them to do their own research. If you or they ever need support the help line for CMS is easy to remember: 1-800-MEDICARE.

Medicaid is a joint federal and state program that helps with medical costs for some people with limited income and resources

Essentially, Medicaid is a national program to provide insurance to the indigent with significant medical conditions. Though the government has a standard poverty definition, different states have varying cut-offs and levels for funding patients' needs. States are the arbiter of Medicaid funds, each with varying program designations, fees, schedules, etc. It serves as a valuable alternative to lack of care for many patients.

Other forms of governmental insurance exist including insurance for Native Americans, Tricare for military families/ governmental employees, and the VA system for veterans. As a resident, your interaction with these forms of care will likely be limited or very structured. Many residencies have rotations at the VA where care for veterans is provided at vastly decreased cost compared to that available in the community.

27.2   Insurance as a Resident

As a house officer, your interactions with insurance will be relatively limited. The majority will occur in the form of approval for components of a patient's in house care or care after discharge. You will potentially need to engage insurance companies for things such as durable medical equipment (so-called DME—think wound vac, or prostheses), approval for placement in a form of rehabilitation facility, or scheduling a case for a patient. Short of these types of approval, when performing in-patient clinical tasks, you will have little inter-action with insurance companies.

When booking cases in a clinic or office, the opposite is true. The majority of hospital admissions on nonemergent basis occur using a process known as "pre-certification." This essentially means that the support staff working for the physi-cian contacts the patient's insurance company and briefly outlines the diagnosis made, the proposed treatment plan, the expected hospital stay, and other questions. Your representa-tive then is given a precertification number. This number is then used to interface with the hospital for that particular hospital visit. All charges to the patient and their insurance company correspond to that precertification number. This process is different in entirely government facilities. Residents themselves are often asked to obtain precertification for large outpatient cases scheduled at VA facilities since the precertification process is entirely internal.

Occasionally, you will want to perform certain procedures or admit patients to the hospital and the insurance carrier will refuse outright or deny coverage for a type of procedure. This usually begins a lengthy and frustrating back-and-forth dia-logue between you and the carrier regarding the need for the procedure. This may go as far as to require not only docu-mentation of the diagnosis for the patient based on test results and exam findings, but also supporting evidence. Often carriers will have you speak with another physician—one employed by the carrier—in order to justify your course of action. This happens frequently when using things "off label" or without FDA approval. The most frequent response by surgeons is to provide documentation as well as several peer reviewed articles with highest-level-available evidence.

The emergent situation supersedes all insurance situations. It should go without saying that doing what is right is always most important. If a patient needs emergent surgery, then get the case done and worry about paying for it later. Should the patient be uninsured, you regardless have an ethical mandate to treat them. It is often a component of the mission of for-profit hospitals to provide a certain percentage of their care as pro-bono/for uninsured patients. Doubtless you have encountered the late night transfer as a resident for an emergent surgical condition that could have been handled with aplomb by the transferring surgeon because the patient failed the "wallet biopsy." This route of action is deplorable as a physician.

27.3   The Uninsured: Your Role

The traditional patients in teaching hospitals and clinics of the past were indigents with little other choice than to go to a facility with inexperienced physicians on call and performing necessary care—at least in the eyes of the public. We know this to be inaccurate. However, you will frequently come across patients without insurance as a part of your training. The treatment of these patients should be same regardless of their insurance status, but this is often not the case. That said, what is the role of the house officer in the care of the uninsured?

First, you must familiarize yourself with the matters of recourse within your community to provide medical coverage for those that have none. Perhaps your state is one that has excellent coverage for the indigent. These programs often take the form of named cards or programs that will be known to the medical community—the nurses working in the clinics are usually the best source of information here. Other times programs are available through the municipal government for enrollment—each large city is different and will have different options. You will know through experiences which of these programs enroll which types of patients.

Your second duty is to help your patients establish insurance if they have none. No one expects a surgery resident to work as hard as you do and spend time filling out paperwork with a patient to apply for insurance. You should however be facile enough with the options to spend 2 or 3 min at the end of an encounter with a patient to explain their options in your community and point them in the correct direction.

27.4   The Affordable Care Act

The ACA, or Obamacare, is a massive piece of legislation passed in March, 2010. The goal of the ACA was to provide coverage for those in America not currently covered by private insurance or governmental insurance. The supplemental goals included: adding young people (under age 26) to their parents' health insurance, the end of denial of coverage for preexisting conditions, cost free preventive care, justification for increased premiums, and a myriad of other goals. While laudable, the bill is a 2,000 page long gargantuan with long standing implications and changes to health care that are only now being implemented. No one knows the effect that the ACA will have on health care in America in the long run. Some believe it will reduce costs by moving the goal of care to preventive medicine. Others believe it will only expand the healthcare market place by insuring a larger number of people. Will these people then consume U.S. health care at a greater rate than the average patient? So many questions remain unanswered.

As a resident, you will sadly have little control over this issue save those actions available to the public at large depending on your feeling about the law itself. Your current best course of action is to keep yourself apprised of changes in the landscape of health care and make plans accordingly. The authors advise you to complete your medical training with fervor and to the best of your ability. If you emerge a well-trained, capable, compassionate physician, patients will flock to you no matter the insurance climate. You are encouraged to become actively involved in local and national politics so that you can be a part of these healthcare decisions.

Chapter 28
Vacations

Your vacation time is precious to you. Do not waste a moment of it. Your body and mind depend on periods of rest. It should be mandatory to get out of town and do something mindless for a few days a year. There is no intention in this chapter to tell you where to go or what to do; however, with a little study and forethought, you will be able to schedule a vacation like the expert you will become.

The following suggestions will assure you that the planning essentials of your vacation will be done in a timely and complete fashion.

- Negotiate the schedule and coverage with your colleagues. Remember, they will have to pick up the slack.
- Schedule your vacation in writing with the department at least 6 weeks in advance.
- Make sure there are no scheduling conflicts with other residents.
- For obvious reasons, and whether or not it is a rule, do not schedule vacations for the 6-week period beginning July 1, or for the month of June.
- Several people should know how to contact you in case of an emergency. Leave your travel plans and destination phone number with the department secretary, your chief resident, and whoever is staying in your home.

L.D. Florman, *The Portable Medical Mentor:*
Training Success, DOI 10.1007/978-3-319-09852-4_28,
© Springer International Publishing Switzerland 2015

- Before you actually leave, call the switchboard and tell them that you will be away, and whom to call in your absence.
- Just before departing, debrief your colleagues about your patients in the hospital as well as any patients with particular problems.
- Complete all of your dictation and medical records.
- Any patients at home with ongoing problems may be told of your departure, and whom to call if necessary.

Here are some additional suggestions:

- Space your vacations throughout the year instead of taking them all at one time.
- Think ahead so that you can combine vacation time with scheduled holidays that fall on Friday or Monday. These will be fairly popular vacation times, so schedule early. Regrettably these travel times will also be more expensive.
- Make vacation reservations at least 3 months in advance (6 months is better).
- For airlines, boats, and hotels, it is a good idea to follow several online discount agencies. You can subscribe to their online mailing lists for cheap fares, rates, and deals. If you see a fare that you can live with, go to the website of the carrier (i.e., Delta Airlines, American Airlines, Hilton Hotels) and determine whether they can beat the price. Don't procrastinate. The fares often change rapidly.
- Package deals (transportation, hotel, food) can save you money.

Chapter 29
Finances

> *"Money is better than poverty, if only for financial reasons."*
>
> — Woody Allen

> *"No matter how rich you become, how famous or powerful, when you die the size of your funeral will still pretty much depend on the weather."*
>
> — Michael Pritchard

No, we are not going to instruct you on how to spend your pittance of a paycheck. Nonetheless, your resident's pay will place you in the middle class of all American taxpayers. A few suggestions taken seriously now just may ease your way through the financial jungle you are bound to have, when you are in a better monetary situation. You will find some of the topics in this chapter very current. Others should be kept in the back of your mind, to use when the occasion arises.

29.1 Medical Malpractice Insurance

This will be purchased for you by the hospital. Two important aspects that you should be concerned with are: Is this a claims *made* or an *occurrence* policy? "Claims made" means that in order to be covered, the claim against you must be filed while

L.D. Florman, *The Portable Medical Mentor:*
Training Success, DOI 10.1007/978-3-319-09852-4_29,
© Springer International Publishing Switzerland 2015

you are insured with that company. In other words, when you leave your residency, you are no longer insured for a claim that was made against you during your residency. One remedy for this is to insist that your next insurer provides (usually at no cost) "*tail coverage.*" This will cover you for acts committed during your residency. The other option is for your hospital to buy you an "occurrence" policy. This will cover you by the hospital's insurance company no matter where you are, or when the suit is filed against you.

Another factor in malpractice insurance is the *limits of coverage*. What is the total amount the insurance company will cover? If your net worth is in the millions, this might be a very important number to know. Recent jury awards have been in the tens of millions of dollars.

Unfortunately, all of this is rather moot, as you have little or no say in the type of policy or coverage amount you are given. Nevertheless, you should attempt to educate yourself on these issues, as malpractice insurance will be required for the rest of your career, and you must eventually become an expert on the subject.

29.2   Life Insurance

If you are given life insurance as part of your resident's employment package, you should inquire about the possibility of extending it when you leave the institution. The earlier in life you are insured, the less premium you will pay. Also, consider purchasing the insurance for the longest possible time, with a fixed premium that can't be increased.

It is a good idea to study the types of life insurance before buying it. But, don't wait too long, as your premium will only increase. It is wise to be careful, because a lot of insurance sales people are scouting for young doctors.

In general, there are two kinds of individual policies, *whole life* and *term*. A term policy is less expensive and has a fixed annual premium for a certain number of years. The coverage, however, stops when you stop paying the premium or the certain number of years has expired. A whole life policy is a good way for a young person to be insured. It is more expensive than a term policy, but part of the premium is invested for you, and you benefit from the interest, which is reinvested for you. This interest amount will eventually pay the premiums, year after year. So, if you have been diligent in paying your premiums in the beginning years, you will be insured at no cost in the later years. You may also borrow against the money in your account.

Purchasing life insurance is very important when needed, but everybody does not need it. The entire subject becomes almost a philosophy of life. Most will agree that it should not be considered a lottery winning for the beneficiaries. If you have children and/or your spouse has a good job, they may not need your insurance money. If you have incurred considerable debt as a result of home loans, car loans, and school loans, insurance money will come in handy for those you leave behind. Remember, life insurance is rather costly, and if it is not necessary, don't buy it. But, before you take this advice, you should check with knowledgeable people. Everybody's situation is different, and the options are endless.

Remember, with life insurance, it pays to start young.

29.3   Disability Insurance

Most residency training programs will purchase a small disability insurance policy for you. If you must pay the premium yourself, you should be aware of the following: Make sure you are covered if you are disabled in your specialty. Or, you might find yourself disabled to do surgery, but not psychiatry. You will also want to know the time period from when you are totally disabled, to when the checks start to arrive. The shorter this lag period, the more the premium. Also, the period of disability covered should last at least until age 64, and premium payment should be suspended during the time of disability.

Usually, the institution-paid-for disability policy is not adequate for the average young professional. You should be able to increase it significantly for a fairly low premium. It could be very worth your while to do that, especially if you have a young family.

29.4   Healthcare Insurance

Most certainly your institution will pay for your healthcare insurance. Be concerned and ask questions about the co-pay, deductibles, prescription drugs, and excluded benefits (like mental illness). The exclusion of mental illness is not acceptable in today's world, where it seems as though more and more doctors are developing addictions, or committing suicide. There is not much you can do about these items short of paying additional premiums. However, it might make sense to consider the expense. You can often opt to add coverage for dental and vision services. They are most often worth the small added expense.

Read your policy carefully for hidden benefits like discounts on eyeglasses, medical devices, medications, etc.

In the years to come, you will become an expert on healthcare insurance, so start now to understand this evolving subject.

29.5   Long-Term Care Insurance

You may be a bit too young to consider long-term care but, again, the younger you are when you buy, the less the premium. It's a good idea to educate yourself on this subject.

29.6   Automobile Insurance

Don't skimp on liability insurance for you and your family. The maximum coverage does not cost much more than the minimum. Don't forget that you are now a doctor and when the other side finds that out, they will go after everything that you own now or will own in the future. There is a type of insurance policy called an *umbrella*. It virtually adds insurance on top of the insurance you already have. For example, if your automobile policy has a liability limit of $500,000, the umbrella could add another $500,000, giving you one million dollars' worth of protection. This same umbrella covers your home owner's insurance, malpractice insurance, and whatever other kind of liability insurance you might have.

29.7   Avoid Unnecessary Debt

It is not a very comfortable feeling to have amassed a lot of debt by the time you are finished with your training. Just when you want to start out fresh in practice, you have a big nut to crack, specifically a lot of interest and principle to pay. You will be enticed to borrow money with very little interest at first, and later for a lot of interest. Don't do it. Purchasing a house or a condominium might be one of the only sane ways of incurring debt at your stage of life. Again, this is going to take a lot of restraint, study, and some expert advice.

Do not incur excessive credit card debt. Live within your means.

29.8   Seeking Expert Financial Advice

Open up a checking account (no fees for small balances, no charge for checks) at a large bank. The bank has experts in every department who will not necessarily have a vested interest in selling you something. They are usually willing to talk, but often will not tell you to do something in particular. Consider them educators. They will be more interested in you when you go into practice or get a good job. For now, they are usually happy to advise you, while waiting for you to get to the "big times."

On the subject of educators, you might discuss any financial decisions you have to make with one of your attendings who you like and trust. Remember, they have been through this already. In the end, it is you who will have to make the final decision, so you had better educate yourself.

29.9   Savings

You will have many years ahead of you to think about saving money. However, because of your relative youth, you have an amazing opportunity to put away a small amount of money in a tax-free savings account, and just let it sit for years, quietly growing. If you can just see your way clear to put at least $200 a month in a Roth IRA, you will be delighted to see what it is worth in 10, 20, or 30 years. The Roth IRA is somewhat of a gift to young people from your Federal government.

29.10   Subscription to a Money Magazine

Immediately subscribe to one of the many money magazines (Money, Kiplinger's, Wall Street Journal, etc.) and read it cover to cover every month. The articles may not interest you today, but they will be salient in the future. You will not only read about current financial events, but you will also see trends in finance, and who knows, you may even be able to talk to friends about your big business prowess. The idea is not to wait until you are in a critical financial situation before you start reading. Educate yourself now.

   You never went into medicine to be burdened with the world of insurance and financial calculations. However, it is or will soon become a sort of parallel profession to you. There is no escaping it, and it cannot be subjugated to others. In the end, you will have to do the best that you can to educate yourself and sort through these incredibly complex subjects.

Chapter 30
Assorted Affairs

30.1 Cameras

A camera is a valuable tool for residents in several specialties:

- To document the extent of injuries.
- To document appropriate preoperative and intraoperative pathology.
- To document postoperative results.
- To document skin lesions and rashes.
- To copy X-rays for presentations.
- To assist in PowerPoint presentations.
- To photograph family and friends.

For those residents and fellows in the specialties dealing with the surgery of appearance (oral-maxillofacial surgery, otolaryngology-head and neck surgery, plastic surgery), a camera is indispensable and should be carried at all times.

At this writing, approximately 85 % of all cameras sold in the United States are digital. There are many digital cameras to choose from and so many variations in options; it will be impossible to sort them out for you in this book. However, you should be aware of some of the important features to look for and learn about.

L.D. Florman, *The Portable Medical Mentor:*
Training Success, DOI 10.1007/978-3-319-09852-4_30,
© Springer International Publishing Switzerland 2015

Consider when purchasing:

- The number of pixels generally refers to the final quality of the picture the camera will produce. The more pixels, the less grainy the picture. It is important to realize that there are other factors that contribute to the final quality, such as monitor quality, photographic paper quality, and projector quality. Pixels are expensive, so there is a limit to the number of pixels you should consider purchasing. Most professional photographers believe that for routine medical photography, 3.5 megapixels is all that you need. You will not see the difference in printed or projected work with more than 3.5 megapixels.
- Digital Zoom vs. Optical Zoom.
- Lenses.
- Single Lens Reflex cameras.
- Batteries should be at least lithium, rechargeable, and you should always have an extra in your bag.
- Storage devices usually consist of minidisks. Most cameras are sold with only a small-sized disk. It will be necessary to purchase a larger one (1 gigabyte) immediately.
- Some cameras have the ability to record video. This feature, although not very useful in medicine, is nice to have. A considerable amount of storage (1 gigabyte) permits several minutes of filming in this mode.
- Software comes with each camera. Make sure that it is compatible with your computer, fairly easy to use, and that it has a rather comprehensive filing system so that you can appropriately organize the hundreds of pictures that you will take.
- The display is a very important feature that deserves mentioning. Not only should it be clear and bright, but it should also swivel so that you can take bird's eye view pictures in the operating room.

Question your attendings and the more senior residents. Ask them what they like and don't like about their cameras.

You should now be getting the idea that purchasing a camera for medical purposes is a very complicated process.

In speaking with sales personnel, you will be able to quickly discern if they know what they are talking about. If they don't, then move on to another store. You might try speaking with the photographer on staff at your hospital or university. They are usually very willing to help.

The camera features in smartphones and tablets are becoming more and more sophisticated. These may be a very valid option.

30.2   Charity

Interns and residents are a poor bunch, or so they think. In reality, they are right in the middle of monetary compensation in the entire country. We all give in the form of free care or indigent care; that is your duty and privilege. Charity is another story. It does not always mean giving money. There are many ways you can be charitable; however, money is often the most needed method, and the least time-consuming for your busy schedule.

Consider a couple of dollars a week to a charity of your choice. Work at a soup kitchen once a month. Volunteer to the Red Cross or Salvation Army once in a while. There are so many ways to give that you will have no trouble finding them or them finding you. Involve your spouse and your children.

30.3   Computers

This is a huge subject, and in another forum, could occupy the space of an entire book. In today's world you must have a computer. Laptop or desktop is up to you. Realize that either will be more than adequate for the needs of most individuals. You should be very discriminating in purchasing this item, and at the same time understand that this will not be the first, second, or even third computer that you will own.

Some things to keep in mind:

• Get the largest screen that you can afford, and have the physical space for. Flat screens are nice and state of the art. The liquid crystal display (LCD) is probably not necessary in a computer monitor, and are more expensive.

• Get the largest hard drive that you can afford.

• Get the most memory that you can afford. Actually, memory affects your speed more than the central processing unit (CPU).

• Don't spend much money on processor speed.

• Make sure that Microsoft Office with PowerPoint is installed.

• If you are able, you should negotiate to have photo editing software (Adobe Photoshop, Ulead, etc.) installed at no charge to you.

• Printers come in all sizes, shapes, and qualities. They all will do the job, and usually will have to be replaced in 1–3 years. A laser printer will be more expensive, but may be worth the extra money in the long term. Aside from the higher quality print, a laser printer will print 1,000 copies for about the same price as an ink-jet printer will print 100 copies.

• An all-in-one printer includes a scanner, which is necessary to have.

• A CD-RW (read/write) is mandatory. A DVD–RW is nice to have.

• Don't fool around with dial-up internet service. Get a DSL or equivalent line, and subscribe to the largest server.

• It is more practical at this stage of your life to buy a named brand computer with matching accessories. It is not a good idea to put together a hybrid computer from a little known manufacturer.

You can spend a lot of time accessorizing your computer setup, but for now, the above suggestions will give you a good start.

30.4   Ethics

It appears that there is a slightly different set of ethics for every job, profession, organization, government, and religion. *Medical Ethics* is described as: "The rules or standards governing the conduct of a person or the conduct of the members of a profession." Truly, the principles of medical ethics were set down by Hippocrates in his "oath," (Chap. 24.2) and if we carefully dissect it, we will be able to answer almost every ethical question that we will encounter. The problem is that so many of our contemporary ethical dilemmas now require an interpretation, often by committee, to the exclusion of the more ancient, simple, practical tenants of the code of ethics.

This subject is huge, often overwhelming, and beyond the scope of this book. For more than 155 years, the American Medical Association's *Code of Medical Ethics* has been the standard and most comprehensive guide to physicians on ethics related issues. It is published on their website, and we commend it to you.

30.5   History

The history of medicine has been well documented for centuries. We learn from those who came before us as well as those who are in our midst. These inquisitive and inventive minds have shaped our profession into what it is today, to say nothing of the countless sick and injured people they have helped through the millennia. So many of the illnesses, procedures, and instruments that we use still bear their names, so it is important that we know who they were, and are, what they did to enrich our specialty, and why they did it.

Do not pass up a name without performing at least a cursory search of the individual. Do not pass up the history sections of the books that you will read about medicine and surgery. Do not be timid about using the names of the great men and women who have made medicine what it is today.

We truly do stand on the shoulders of giants.

30.6   Hobbies

Of course you don't have time for hobbies. Make the time! Hobbies do not include sports activities. Hobbies are just for you, to think about, play at, nurture, and enjoy. Some suggestions:

- Bonsai tree growing
- Knitting, crocheting
- Drawing
- Raising cockroaches
- Aquariums
- Racing mice
- Investing your wealth

What we are endeavoring to say is that your entire life need not revolve around medicine. Diversify and enrich yourself.

30.7   Left Handedness

Society is not sympathetic to the left-handed person. Surgery is a right-handed profession. All of the instruments and equipment we use are for righted-handed surgeons. It is possible to have left-handed instruments, but most lefties find them awkward to use, as they have, for the most part, adapted to the right hand way of life from a very early time.

The main reason for these few words about handedness is to tell those left-handed students in surgery that they should not use this impediment as a crutch. Don't complain about it and don't make excuses for it. It is probably not a good idea to teach yourself to be ambidextrous, as your brain is already too well adjusted to left handedness. Just do the best that you can do, and realize that you are in good company with the likes of Leonardo da Vinci, Beethoven, Michelangelo, Ben Franklin, Isaac Newton, Albert Einstein, Charlie Chaplin, Picasso, and the infamous Jack the Ripper.

30.8   Library and Filing System

It is never too early to start building your own, personal library. You have saved some of the important books from medical school, and that is a good start. Books on the basic sciences should be kept forever. The standard textbooks can be quite expensive, but are very necessary to have. If there is a particular book that you must have, and cannot afford, you might ask one of the pharmaceutical representatives to purchase it for you. You should ask the industry representatives whether there are any particular books which they routinely give to residents. Always be on the lookout for antique books and books of historical interest.

Throughout your residency, you will accumulate papers, brochures, handouts, reprints, etc., which most often will result in stacks of papers and ultimately will end up in the trash. Much of this "stuff" is good to have for reference when the times arise. Start now by purchasing a box of color file folders. Place these documents in appropriately labeled folders, and save them forever. Or, scan them into an electronic file system. It will make your life a little more orderly. You can easily refer to them when necessary. Some of them will have a historical value in years to come.

30.9   Missions

During your training, you may have the opportunity to participate in a medical mission to some underserved area on this planet. If at all possible, do not pass up these opportunities. In fact, seek them out. Your chief will most likely be proud to permit you to go, and you will benefit not only educationally, but with a real sense of having done something good. The expenses of some missions are paid for by various agencies. More often than not, you will have to pay.

30.10   Political Action Committees

It seems a little distant to be thinking of politics at a time like this in your training, but, as much as we may not approve, both local and national politics is a part of medicine today, and we just have to get used to it. It seems that physicians and politicians do not speak the same language, do not see the same things in their constituencies, and do not have the same goals for health care. Today, there are many physicians who hold prestigious positions in our government, and who speak for us. It is up to you to continue this medical education of the politicians and to place them in positions of governmental power. Go to the AMA website and educate yourself about this important subject.

Chapter 31
The Transition: Part 2

"If you limit your choices only to what seems possible or reasonable, you disconnect yourself from what you truly want, and all that is left is a compromise."

—Robert Fritz

31.1 Introduction

Transitioning out of your training program is a complicated and lengthy procedure. In reality it starts with your graduation from medical school. This chapter should be read and digested by not only the resident or fellow who is finishing his training but also those just beginning their training, as the preparation for this transition really began when you decided to become a doctor. This is, or will be, the culmination of everything that you have worked so hard for, and your every action should be directed to that day when you will assume the responsibility for making the medical decisions, for where you and your family will live, and precisely how you will want to practice your new skills. Many of the aspects in this decision-making process will evolve quite naturally and automatically as time goes on. Your goals may go through several changes as your ability and mind develops, and your needs change. This is a very healthy process. However, you must start preparing and positioning yourself very early on for the numerous life-changing events that are in store for you.

L.D. Florman, *The Portable Medical Mentor:*
Training Success, DOI 10.1007/978-3-319-09852-4_31,
© Springer International Publishing Switzerland 2015

This section of the book is meant to be only a primer to facilitating your transition from the rather sheltered life of training to the certainly complex life in the real world of medicine. You will have to digest a plethora of information in a short period of time, becoming an expert on subjects which you have not yet heard of. Throughout this necessary ordeal, you must not lose sight of your primary mission; practice good medicine, take care of your family and yourself, and be a good citizen.

31.2   The Start

The practice of medicine is a passion. For some, general medicine (family practice) satisfies that passion very well, but for others, for one reason or another, a specialty meets the need for fulfillment. For some, the full training in one of the major specialties is not enough, and more specialized training can be had in the form of a fellowship. Your choices following residency are numerous:

- Fellowship training
- Private practice

    - Solo
    - Group

        Single specialty
        Multispecialty

- Academia
- Another specialty
- Additional degree
- Administration
- Retire

Each possibility has many alternatives, which become a matter of investigation and elimination. It is not unusual for a person to choose one route, and following analysis, eliminate it, and select another. In reality, there are no rules for choosing. It just seems to come with experience and a great deal of patience and desire.

It is acceptable not to have chosen your final goal early in the process, but some day you will have to weigh all of the variables and reach a firm decision on what you want to do with the rest of your life. So many factors will determine your decision that it is impossible to advise you in this book. In the end, it is often a very difficult decision to make, and it is one that should never be made by default. In other words, don't choose a less-than-perfect avenue for the future just because the other avenues may be worse.

You can be assured that your final decision will most likely be correct if once you have made that decision, you stop debating the issue, and put your entire self into your new choice.

31.2.1 Fellowship Training

Fifteen to twenty percent of those completing one of the high profile residencies will seek additional training in the form of a fellowship. Choosing a certain fellowship position depends on precisely what you are looking for in postgraduate education, who is in charge of the fellowship program, and in what part of the country you want to spend 6 months or a year. Fellowship should be considered if:

- There is a particular expertise that you want to acquire.
- Your training was deficient in a particular subject.
- You want to bide time while waiting for a practice opportunity.

Fellowships are offered by institutions and by private individuals. Although there are lists of fellowships available, and many of them advertise positions in the journals, the best way to learn about them is from your attendings and your chief. They are able to make recommendations based on their experience and knowledge of the principal individuals in the fellowship programs.

Acceptance to most fellowship programs is highly competitive, and the ACGME matching program does not apply to many of them. You should start the process of applying at the very earliest time permitted. Remember, only the best letters of introduction and recommendation will help you. Telephone calls or candid comments by your chief or attendings will embellish your application.

An interview will certainly be required and will likely be the most important aspect of your application. Be assured the interviewer will be very experienced and able to pick up on the nuances of every word that you say. Be yourself. Be relaxed. Don't practice answers. Don't brag. Just permit your education, desire, and personality to shine through.

This application process must reflect every aspect of your life and persona to date. If you have been an exemplary student, you should not have much trouble seeking the most appropriate fellowship.

31.2.2   Private Practice

Approximately 80 % of residents and fellows completing their training will choose private practice. Generally, in making this very important decision, you should consider the following two questions, and strictly adhere to their order of importance:

1. Where do you and your spouse/significant other want to live?
   This is the most important question, and many factors enter into this decision (i.e., geographical location, climate, schools, family, leisure opportunities, ease of travel to and from that location, homes, crime rate). It is essential that your spouse, fiancé, or significant other is in total agreement. Keep in mind that this, like your decision to enter the medical profession, is a lifetime decision, and will be very disruptive to change.
2. Where is the need?
   Why place yourself in a situation where there is an overabundance of specialists like you? Oh yes, you are better than them. Better looking. Better trained. More likeable. None of that counts. If the area is overcrowded, you will probably not thrive.

3. Solo, group, multispecialty, or clinic?
   This decision will be based on the type of person you are, your ultimate goals in the practice of medicine, the opportunities available to you, and whether you desire to be your own boss, work for others, or a combination of the two.

   There are many resources available to help you in this decision, notably, the American Medical Association and your specialty society. We cannot advise you as to the type of practice, because of the complexity of the variables and the continuous changes in each possibility. These many factors will become very apparent to you as you begin to sort out what is available.

Considering practice options can begin as early as your first year, but should not occupy much of your thoughts until well into your last year. By January of your last year, you should know where you are going, be comfortable with the people involved, and be far along in the negotiation phase. Always leave ample time and have stand-by options, should these negotiations break down. Under no circumstances should you force yourself into any kind of practice as a last ditch measure.

Generically speaking, preparation for practice opportunities coincides with the beginning of your residency training. All of the things that we have discussed in this book will now embellish your chances of getting the best fellowship, or attracting the most worthy private practices. Or, these same "things" can come back to haunt you. This would be a good time to again read Chap. 3. Now, you will have to demonstrate to others, usually outside of your training program, that you are the appropriate choice. You will also have to depend on those in your institution for kind words and helpful suggestions. If there is someone who you did not get along well with, you can be assured that he will be contacted for a candid discussion of your character. Your entire education, your whole persona, and your fondest dreams all come to this convergence point in time. Repetition is in order:

Be **honest** (with yourself and others).
Be **kind** (with yourself and others) (it costs you nothing).

Be **humble**.
Be **prepared**.

31.2.3   Academia

Academic careers can be very satisfying and must be seriously considered when deciding what to do with your life. The rewards are numerous; however they carry a totally different set of problems than private practice.

Interestingly, most interviewees for residency and fellowship positions will, when asked, about their future plans, will state that they want academics. In fact, only 7 % will ultimately go into academic medicine.

Pros

– Intellectually rewarding.
– Relatively stable.
– Opportunity to advance in rank.
– Established practice.
– No initial financial obligation.
– Interns and residents to assist you.
– Research and writing opportunities.
– Camaraderie.
– Cutting edge in medicine.
– Opportunity for innovation.
– Coverage.
– Large institution benefits.
– A good jump-off point to private practice.

Cons

– You are not your own boss.
– May not be as financially rewarding.
– You do not choose your partners.
– You must perform academically to stay in.
– Numerous meetings.
– A small voice in a large crowd.

31.3   The Search

Many practice offers appear fortuitously, but it is up to you to keep your eyes and ears open and take a proactive role in at least superficially investigating all possible practice opportunities. A good place to begin your search is with your attendings and chief. These discussions should take place "by appointment," not in hallways or over the operating table. Knowing your abilities, capabilities, and temperament, they are in the best position to advise you and attempt to match you with an appropriate opportunity.

Continuously monitor the classified advertisements in your specialty society's periodic journals, the *Journal of the American Medical Association*, the throw-away journals and magazines, and the internet medical bulletin boards. There will be booths at the large national meetings and conferences with representatives of companies who make it their business to find jobs for young doctors. You should make yourself known at each. It is a very good idea to go to at least one national meeting a year (even if you have to pay). This is where you will network for the future. There are medical headhunters who will eventually seek you out; it is not a good idea to wait for this to happen, as the timing most certainly will not be appropriate.

31.3.1   The Decision

We hope that this will be the last major career decision that you will have to make. Sometimes the decision of what to do following graduation comes very fortuitously, not infrequently with a casual offer of a practice opportunity. Sometimes the same decision-making process is very painful and disruptive to your life. Regardless, it pays to take your time with the process, be thorough in your investigations, and don't get yourself into any situation, or become associated with any person, until you are completely comfortable. At this point, you have not obligated yourself to any definitive decision; that is a long way off. If you are not comfortable with future negotiations, you must courteously go back to your search options and consider this false start as a lesson in business. Once you have come to a tentative conclusion, and there is an offer on the table, it is time to start the rather lengthy, sometimes expensive, always difficult, process of actually making the deal.

31.3.2   The Investigation

To this point, you have done everything correctly, and now it behooves you to expend a considerable amount of effort into meticulously investigating the opportunity possibilities you have chosen. This is the most important exercise in the process. An offer has been made, albeit casual and in general terms. Much discussion has occurred, and you and your future partner (practitioner, group, university, clinic, hospital) have agreed in principal that you are, or could be, compatible, have similar goals, thoughts of practice, ethics, work principles, and that now you should proceed with the details. The verbal agreements that you have both made should now be put into a formal written contract. Read it carefully. It should agree in essence with all that you have discussed. If it does not, you must call your future partner and iron out the problems. This is best done in person, by telephone, and not email. If the major points of contention cannot be worked out, then it is time to respectfully and hastily begin looking for another opportunity. If the issues are minor, then work them out. Remember, a good partnership is like a good marriage; give and take.

Once the contract looks good, you must take it to an attorney of your choosing who is very familiar with employment contracts for physicians. He will dissect it, explain to you the possible pitfalls, and probably rewrite parts of it. He may even reinvent it to the point where it becomes untenable to your future partner. Attorneys have a tendency to make contracts so correct that the human and practical elements become secondary. It will be up to you, in consultation with your attorney, to decide what is important to you, and worth the fight and what is not important, or not worth making issues which could only antagonize.

A "noncompete" clause will most likely be included in any contract that you receive. It will be better if you can negotiate your way out of it, or at least have it wear off after a reasonable period of time, such as 1 year. Noncompetes (sometimes called "covenant not to compete") protect the principle entity from your gathering his practice and going into competition across the street. Once signed, they are very difficult, if not impossible to revoke. Most states will uphold a noncompete clause under any circumstance, and most contracts will contain one. For this reason, it is good to take your time and be as sure as you are able that this proposed partnership is right for you.

Additional items that must be addressed and carefully evaluated in a contract will be:

- Remuneration
- Term of the contract
- Buy-ins, buy-outs
- Partnership tract
- Malpractice insurance (don't forget tail coverage)
- Disability insurance
- Life insurance
- Expense apportioning
- Special equipment, instrument you might need
- Work apportioning
- Vacations
- Exit from practice strategies for you and for your partner

Some items that may not be part of the contract but are important to know:

- Staff support and who pays for it.
- Auto lease or expense.
- Signage.
- Marketing expenses.
- Routine inspection of the accounting books.

In the short space of this book, it is difficult to identify all of the idiosyncrasies of a contract between doctors or between doctors and entities. We can only say that there are many, and that professional, unemotional, detached help is required.

31.3.3   Due Diligence

Before signing on the dotted line, it is a good idea to take a time-out for a few days to 3 or 4 weeks and to just:

• Reflect on what you have accomplished.
• Compare your dreams to the realities that are about to take place.
• Assure yourself that you are not just settling for second best.
• Make sure that the lofty goals that you have set for yourself will be satisfied.
• Be peaceful that you are making the correct decisions for your present and future families.

31.3.4   Obligations

This chapter on transitions would not be complete without reminding you of your departing obligations to your present training program. Here is a quick checklist:

• Work until the last day.
• Do not save your vacations until June.
• Make sure your dictations are up to date.
• Visit the medical records department just prior to the end.
• Leave your forwarding home phone number, business phone number, fax number, cellular number, home address, and business address with the department secretary.
• Clean out your locker, and return the key to the proper person.
• Make a special point of going around the hospital and thanking people who have been a part of your life on your way up.
• Say a special farewell and thank you to your chief and your attendings. Ask them if you may communicate with them in the future.

31.4   The Beginning

Your mentors have finished instructing you in the fine art of the practice of medicine, and how to behave as a physician. The rest is up to you. There are no books to show you how to comport yourself in practice. On June 30th, you were a resident or fellow. On July 1st, all of a sudden you are a "real doctor." Very simply, you only need to practice the principles of good medicine that you have learned, and strictly adhere to the basic rules: be honest, be humble, be kind, and be prepared. Oh yes, there are now two more rules: be proud and be happy.

Chapter 32
The Mentor's Wrap-Up

"I imagine the life of a surgeon can be very rewarding…"
"Obviously you have saved the lives of many people…"
"Is that what led you to become a surgeon?"
"No, I just liked the little green booties!"

— Peanuts

Mentoring students, interns, residents, and fellows is an enriching, enlightening, and satisfying avocation, made possible to only a few of us fortunate enough to be permitted to work with today's bright and dedicated physicians of the future. I am certain that I can take the liberty of speaking for all of us mentors and advisors, and for you as well, the mentors of tomorrow, who will be the standard torchbearers of learning, teaching, researching, and practicing the flower of all professions….MEDICINE.

What follows is the essence of this book. Live by these doctrines, and you will certainly be the pride of our profession:

- You owe a debt of gratitude to each of your patients: good, bad, kind, evil, young, old, clean, dirty, friendly, mean, smelly, happy, angry, calm, violent. If it weren't for them, you would have nobody to learn from. Somehow, in some way, you must show your gratitude.

L.D. Florman, *The Portable Medical Mentor:* 195
Training Success, DOI 10.1007/978-3-319-09852-4_32,
© Springer International Publishing Switzerland 2015

- Have great respect for your teachers; all of them, even the ones you do not like or trust. You learned something from every one of them.
- Never fail to pay attention to your parents, siblings, spouse, children, and friends. It makes you a better person. They were with you on the way up. They will stay by your side on the way down.
- Make every effort to stay healthy in your body and in your mind.
- Keep humor in every aspect of your life.

On the subject of "joking around" about patients, a famous neurosurgeon lamented to me one day that his specialty exposed him to unimaginable and incomparable human tragedies and experiences. When he would find himself laughing or joking at something that was really not funny, he would tell those around him that it was not out of disrespect, ignorance, or malice, but that the only other option was to internalize it and then go home and spend the rest of the day and night in his closet.

- Be compassionate to your patients, to your very soul.

The following aphorisms were compiled by the late Dr. Eugene Kilgore, a hand surgeon, and are known as Kilgoreisms. They are very salient today:

- You can take a lifetime to establish a reputation, and lose it in a day.
- Think, "us," "our," not "me," "I."
- Think, "What can I do to help," not, "That's not my job."
- You have to give to get.
- Don't be reluctant to say, "I don't know."
- Be willing to learn from everyone, especially your patients.
- Run it by one who has been there before, especially if he/she has gray hairs.
- Technique comes naturally or is rapidly learned by most, but judgment takes time and experience.
- Seasoned judgment is the cumulative product of episodes of bad judgment.

- Don't hesitate to delegate to a subordinate colleague, and in them never be intolerant of honest mistakes.
- Responsibility brings out the best in anyone, and breeds early maturity.
- Only do for your patients what you would be willing to have done for yourself.
- Beware of advising "Nothing else has worked, so we'd better operate."
- Surgery is *injury*, and the adage "if you can't cut, you can't cure it," no longer applies.
- Don't practice by intimidation.
- You don't own your patient.
- Encourage a second opinion.
- If a patient would rather go to someone else, encourage it.
- Don't belittle the previous practitioner. Remember that you, too, are not perfect.
- Simplicity is predictable, complexity isn't.
- If you let the patient have sufficient time to tell you in detail what is wrong and how it came about, you will find out what ails him and determine what to do for him.
- Don't be a cookbook physician and surgeon. Improvise and adapt.
- Practice good medicine, not defensive medicine.
- Keep detailed records.
- All patients are not created equally, but all count equally.
- Don't be complacent. Your reputation rests on the success of your treatment of your last patient.
- Man's greatest sin is rationalization of his avoidable errors and crimes of omission and commission.
- Practice medicine as an art, not a science.
- Keep skid chains on your tongue; always say less than you think. How you say it often counts more than what you say.
- Never let an opportunity pass to say a kind and encouraging thing to or about somebody. Praise good work done, regardless of who did it. If criticism is needed, criticize helpfully, never spitefully.

- Be interested in others, in their pursuits, their welfare, their homes, and families. Let everyone you meet, however humble, feel that you regard him/her as one of importance.
- Be cheerful. Keep the corners of your mouth turned up. Hide your pains, worries, and disappointments under a smile. Laugh at good stories and learn to tell them.
- Preserve an open mind on all debatable questions. Discuss, but not argue. It is a mark of superior minds to disagree and yet be friendly.
- Let your virtues speak for themselves and refuse to talk of another's vices. Make it a rule to say nothing of another unless it is something good.
- Be careful of another's feelings. Wit and humor at the other fellow's expense are rarely worth the effort.
- Pay no attention to ill-natured remarks about you. Be assured that nobody will believe them. Disordered nerves and a bad digestion are common causes of backbiting.
- Don't be too anxious about what you believe is due you. Do your work, be patient, and keep your disposition sweet. Forget self and you will be rewarded.

Being a mentor is not difficult, and in fact takes no effort at all. One only needs to selflessly impart Dr. Kilgore's knowledge in a gracious way to an eager student. So, who gets more out of it, the mentor or the mentored? The answer lies with Dr. Kilgore's final piece of advice:

The road to success lies in meeting responsibility with an open inquisitive mind, imagination, and hard work, tempered with humility, kindness, fidelity, time for play, the arts, family, as well as a good laugh. The lasting measure of success is how much remains after you have gone, that continues to be of value to others.

Chapter 33
Epilogue

Experience is something you obtain only after you need it.

Moore's Law of Combat.

I was asked, by the author, to write this epilogue after giving a lecture entitled "What I Wish I Knew When I Started My First Attending Surgeon Position." Only being 6 years into practice, some of the elder statesmen of the department (including the author of this book!) said I was still only in the beginning of my practice of surgery and still had a lot to learn. They were completely correct. I still am learning every day from my friends, colleagues, and patients, but I have learned a lot in the past few years. As I look back and look forward on my career as an academic surgeon I can only offer this small sliver of advice to those who will soon be physicians and possibly surgeons.

First, regardless of whatever field of medicine you choose to study, find a mentor. Manuscripts, such as this, go a long way towards providing you with a good foundation of practical knowledge upon which to build your education and career. However, nothing compares to the role a good mentor can play in your life. Their sagacious advice can go beyond simple exchanges of information. A good mentor can act as a confidant and friend and can help to shepherd you away from

L.D. Florman, *The Portable Medical Mentor:*
Training Success, DOI 10.1007/978-3-319-09852-4_33,
© Springer International Publishing Switzerland 2015

the pitfalls which lay in front of all of us who pursue medicine as a career.

Regarding the importance of mentorship you need only look at your own career choice. Why did you go into surgery, or why did you choose medicine in the first place? Surveys from the late 1990s and early 2000s show that mentorship played a vitally important role in the choice of specialty training and decision to enter any particular residency in over 2/3 of the respondents. Other studies have shown that faculty members who identify a mentor report feeling more confident than their peers, and report a higher job satisfaction than those who do not identify a primary mentor. Is there someone who has influenced you?

Identifying a mentor isn't always easy though. Serendipity can play a role but it shouldn't be the primary driver. Nothing this important should be left to chance! As Thomas Jefferson said, "I am a great believer of luck and I find that the harder I work, the more I have of it." As a mentee, spend time finding someone in your institution that has had a track record of developing students and residents. Find someone who has an interest in your ideas and time to work with you. Find someone with your best interests at heart. It may be more than one person. You may have a mentor for research and a different one for clinical training, but most importantly find someone who challenges you daily to be better.

Aside from finding a mentor, you should realize that your training will never end. In Outliers, Malcolm Gladwell identifies the concept of 10,000 h to master a subject. His basic theory is that you need to spend 10,000 actually doing something in order to really be a master. In this book he gives example after example of this idea. Now we can apply this to medical training as well. First, let's assume that you work 80 h/week for 48 weeks a year during training. That's 3,840 h a year learning to be a doctor. In 3 years you will make 10,000 h. Congratulations, you are a really good doctor! Now, let's look at actual time in surgery. Let's assume you will complete your residency with about 1,000 major cases in the role of surgeon. This leaves you a lot of work left to do at the end of residency! Be ready to continue to learn and work hard because based on a recent survey it will take you between 6 and 8 years out from residency to get all 10,000 h.

Learn to be a team player. The old mantra of "Trust no one" really doesn't work anymore in modern medicine. More and more physicians are part of a larger team treating a patient. Learn how to work with others and learn how to lead a team to get the best outcomes possible for the patients. Communicate frequently and consistently with those around you and accept that everyone on the team has an equal voice. That can be difficult for physicians sometimes, particularly surgeons, but it's important to admit when someone may know more than you and accept their advice. Every chance you get—look for ways to help your fellow residents/students. Before you leave for the day, call the other interns and ask them if there is anything you can do to help them. It's the golden rule of residency— Help them the way you'd like to be helped.

That being said I like to live by two rules within the hospital. The first is, "Delegate action, not responsibility." You can ask someone to do something, but it is still your job to make sure it gets done. The responsibility for a task never changes! As an attending surgeon I might let you do portions of an operation, but it is still my responsibility to make sure you do them correctly. The second rule I learned from Ronald Reagan. In the late 1980s while working on US–Russian relations Ronald Reagan used the phrase, "Trust, but verify" to describe his relationship with the Russians. Accept that information given to you in the hospital is reliable and given to you with the patient's best interests at heart, but make sure the information is correct. Check other sources, do additional research, and this will allow you to build trust in those around you and in yourself.

Set priorities in your life and your career. Find what is most important to you and stand by that whatever the cost. As you move through residency remember you are an exciting, hardworking, intelligent breath of fresh air in most of the hospitals/organization you will be working in…and they will kill you trying to harness that potential. You will be assigned all kinds of projects and meetings that may or may not be in line with your priorities. If they aren't, learn to say no—do it with a smile, do it pleasantly, do it unapologetically—but do it. You won't do yourself or your organization any good if you are spread too thin and unable to accomplish any of the tasks or projects assigned to you.

You are going to want to prove yourself. We all do; learn to do it the right way. Don't take on challenges you are sure to fail while trying to establish yourself at your institution. As an example, don't take on massively complex cases or difficult diagnostic challenges sure to have numerous complications in your first year out of practice. No one will remember that Mr. X had horrible comorbidities and poor health prior to coming under your care, but they will remember that Mr. X had numerous complications and was in the ICU for months following your care. Work hard, always be available, be courteous, and build up a bank of good will within your institution so that when that inevitable complication does arise it will be an aberration not the norm because you are a "good doctor/surgeon."

There is a difference between a complication and a mistake. You will have both happen to you if you are involved in medicine. Complication can be unavoidable and it is important to discuss these with your patients ahead of time if possible. You can do everything right and still have a complication. Also remember that everyone makes mistakes. Learn from them, accept them, vow to not make the same mistake again and move on. Dwelling on mistakes can take its toll on even the most experienced surgeon/physician. You have a great responsibility as a physician but you are still human.

The internet can be your best friend or worse enemy. There are a multitude of great internet sites that help with your medical education. There are great websites for patient education, with fantastic diagrams and videos that can help you explain things and educate the patient more effectively. There is also a lot of junk. Remember Uncle Bob can have website detailing his anecdotal experience with a disease that is as flashy as the National Cancer Institute's patient information site. Know what you are looking at and know what you are looking for when you get online.

Interns/students have a huge amount of paper/computer work (some might refer to this as "scut" work) that needs to be done. It's easy to get lost in the trees and miss the forest. It's too easy to gather the data, write the notes, and wait for someone else (attending, senior resident, etc.) to develop the plan. But that cheats you of your best learning experience; force yourself to pretend that you are the only doctor seeing the patient. What would you do next? If you are ordering a drug, what are the side effects you might see? If you are ordering a test, what do you expect it to show? Formulate a plan. Your attendings (residents) won't always agree with the plan, but that is OK. You can then figure out why theirs is different, what did they see that you didn't.

Call your referring doctors. Call in your consultants and call those who you consult. The medical chart is not always the best way to pass information between treating physicians. Slow down when talking to patients particularly when you are describing a procedure. You have spent hundreds of thousands of dollars on an education and have been at this for years and you barely understand the words that are coming out of your mouth, how do you think Mr. Morales feels? Take time with your patients; enjoy that part of your job.

Finally, remember, have fun in whatever you do. Our profession with all of its regulations, checklists, protocols, and pitfalls is immensely rewarding. We are privileged to see both the miraculous and the terrifying every day. We get to experience what the entire world has to offer at the bedside of our patients. There are immense changes coming to medicine and you should be a part of them because you will be affected by them. It will be difficult: they will sometimes get in the way of taking care of people and they will frustrate you. However, at the end of the day, after all the inane clicky boxes and infinite forms there is a real power in what we do for people. Never lose sight of that.

Jason Smith M.D., PhD.

Appendix A: Commonly Used Web-Based Sites

Medicine in General

World Health Organization
Center for Disease Control
National Library of Medicine (Medline)
WebMD
Mdlinx
Ovid (Journals on line, through library)
HIPAA information

Web-Based Organizations

American Board of Medical Specialties (ABMS)
Accreditation Council for Graduate Medical Education (ACGME)
National Board of Medical Examiners (NBME)
Liaison Committee on Medical Education (LCME)
United States Medical Licensing Examination (USMLE)
Educational Council for Foreign Medical Graduates (ECFMG)
American Medical Association (AMA)
Joint Commission on Accreditation of Hospitals (JCAH)

L.D. Florman, *The Portable Medical Mentor:*
Training Success, DOI 10.1007/978-3-319-09852-4,
© Springer International Publishing Switzerland 2015

Computer Search Engines

Google
Lycos
Metacrawler
Yahoo

PDA

Freeware palm
PDAmd
Epocrates
Avantgo

Travel

MapQuest (maps, directions)
Cheap Tickets (discounter)
ETN (a lot of information)
Expedia (discounter)
Last Minute Travel (last minute)
Hotwire (deals)
Lowest Airfare (discounter)
Orbitz (discounter)
Priceline (fares auction)
Qixo (discounter)
Side Step (deals)
Site 59 (last minute deals)
Sky Auction (fares auction)
Travelocity (discounter)
CNN Travel (travel guide)
Lonely Planet (travel guides)
Fodor's (travel guide)
U.S. State Department Travel Warnings

Finance

Motley Fool
Charles Schwab
Silicon Investor
Yahoo Financial

Appendix B: Books of Interest

Social Media in Clinical Practice, Bertalan Mesko, Springer
  Publications
Gordon's Guide to the Surgical Morbidity and Mortality Conference,
  Leo A. Gordon, M.D. (Hanley & Belfus, Inc., Mosby)

L.D. Florman, *The Portable Medical Mentor:*   209
Training Success, DOI 10.1007/978-3-319-09852-4,
© Springer International Publishing Switzerland 2015